ASCENT FROM CHAOS

Ascent

FROM

Chaos

A PSYCHOSOMATIC
CASE STUDY

PETER E. SIFNEOS

.

HARVARD UNIVERSITY PRESS

CAMBRIDGE, MASSACHUSETTS

1964

TO THE MEMORY OF

MY FATHER

πᾶν μέτρον ἄριστον

PREFACE

IN THIS BOOK I shall describe the case history of one of my patients, a man to whom I am indebted for providing me with a most extraordinary experience. It is the story of an adult who suffered from ulcerative colitis, who was emotionally ill, and who was allowed to depend totally upon his therapist. It is an unusual story, and because of this a few irrelevant facts have been altered so that the patient will remain unrecognizable and confidences will not be violated. These alterations, however, in no way affect the truth of the basic observations on my patient's physical and mental illness.

The source of my material is mainly the collection of my own personal notes, recorded sometimes during or after my interviews, and my recollections of the many day and night encounters I had with this patient. Occasionally it was difficult to take notes. At times it was impossible; yet these were also the times I remember most clearly. It seems that almost every word that was exchanged remains vividly inscribed in my mind. Innumerable discussions with the nurses, the dietitians, the occupational therapist, and my medical, surgical, and psychiatric colleagues helped me in the understanding of this patient and added greatly to the richness of the original material. In all essential matters, I have tried to quote directly from my notes. In some ways these notes may appear naive and my recollections biased, but it should be kept in mind that this history recounts my experience when I was a young and unsophisticated psychiatric resident, treating my most difficult patient.

I wish to express my gratitude to Dr. Stanley Cobb, my

teacher and Chief of Service at that time, for allowing me to carry on such a highly unorthodox procedure, for his support throughout this most difficult period in my professional experience, and for his great kindness in writing the foreword to this book. Dr. Carl Binger's unflinching encouragement that I write the book, and his assistance and valuable comments, are deeply appreciated. I want to thank Dr. Erich Lindemann, my present Chief of Service, for his interest in the treatment of my patient. Acknowledgment is due for his help and support to Dr. Alfred Ludwig, who supervised my work at the time.

I am indebted to Dr. John Nemiah, for his cordial and ready cooperation and for his many helpful suggestions, and to Drs. Charles Clay, Gregory Rochlin, George Talland, Stephen Lorch, and Robert Cserr for their interest and constructive criticism. To Cora Holbrook, whose devoted editorial help made this book readable, I also want to express my appreciation.

Peter E. Sifneos, M.D.

Boston
March 1964

CONTENTS

A GOOD REPORTER of clinical observations always makes a lasting contribution to medicine. We may read about a disease in textbooks, in summarizing journals, and in statistical analyses, but in ten years these all will be dusty and, in twenty years, buried. A conscientious, detailed, and interesting report of even a single case is like a fine portrait; we can return to it again and again when we wish to understand. Its helpfulness is in depth rather than in breadth of view. This is the kind of help the psychotherapist often needs when he turns to the literature for aid in solving a clinical problem. I can wholeheartedly recommend any physician or surgeon responsible for treating a case of ulcerative colitis to read the therapeutic saga here presented by Dr. Sifneos. All students and practitioners of psychiatry, moreover, can get from this book an understanding of what went on between patient and doctor, a private world rarely revealed in medical literature.

The story of Tom's illness is told in eleven chapters, with a final one devoted to discussion. The story stands on its own facts; the discussion is of necessity sometimes speculative and controversial. Dr. Sifneos has approached it with modesty and simplicity. He gives three psychological explanations of how anaclitic therapy may work: the usual one, and two others that are original and somewhat alarming. He does not recommend this therapy as a practicable type of treatment for mental illness or ulcerative colitis. He demonstrates that, in an emergency, when patient and doctor are helpless, it may be a lifesaving procedure. It is thirty-four years since Cecil D. Murray first described the

emotional factors in ulcerative colitis which he observed in
a patient at the Presbyterian Hospital in New York. He was
so far ahead of his colleagues in his thinking that little attention was given to his admirable paper, but in recent years
his findings have been amply substantiated by others, notably
George E. Daniels in New York and Erich Lindemann in
Boston. This book by Dr. Sifneos, however, is not merely
corroborative. It is a remarkable documentation of much
that was theoretical. Where some authors speak of "incor-
poration," Tom tells us in his own words how he thought he
had taken a hated woman into his body and how she was
tearing his guts out!

Much has been written about anaclitic treatment and per-
missiveness. To say the least, it is difficult to arrange and
carry through such a regime on a psychiatric ward, because
so many persons can be upset by one demanding patient.
This is the conventional and practical way of looking at
the problem, but it is superficial. When one has read this
book, he will see that the doctor who carries out anaclitic
therapy becomes so deeply involved and sacrifices so much
that the troubles of the nurses, fellow patients, staff members, and chief of service appear trivial in comparison. The
therapist has to get down to the level of thinking of the
patient, suffering with him and giving up for a time his
own way of life. By this great caring for his patient he may
succeed when things seem hopeless. If so, he has not only
done a great deal for the patient, but has gone through what
Dr. Sifneos calls "a unique and profound life experience."

When Tom was asked by the author for permission to
record and publish the case, he said, "Doc, you must write
your side of it because it is the scientific side, and it must be
known, but please make it sound human. Don't put in big
words that are hard to understand. Make it alive. Try to
show to people what it's like to be in hell and how there is

a way of getting out, and most important of all please write about the two of us." Dr. Sifneos promised to try, and he has succeeded to an extraordinary degree; the story of this journey through the valley of the shadow is deeply human; no big words are used; and it certainly reveals that two persons were struggling together. To those who think that psychiatrists sit in their offices and give advice to patients, this book will be a revelation.

Critics of modern medicine point out that the burden on the practicing physician is so great that he is always in a hurry, finds it impossible to give support by being readily accessible, and has not enough time to give comfort by quiet understanding. Certainly the great technological advances of the last decades have put a great burden on practitioners. To the credit of psychiatry, however, let it be said that more and more emphasis is put on teaching the student to sit and listen (uninterrupted by telephone or secretary) to human stories expressed in the patient's own way. The understanding physician has not disappeared. The reader of this account of Tom's illness will perhaps not despair of finding a compassionate doctor. What is more, he will see evidence presented in this book of a relationship between doctor and patient that not only comforts but heals.

Stanley Cobb, M.D.

ASCENT FROM CHAOS

THE PATIENT to be described in this study suffered from ulcerative colitis, the onset of which was closely related to a psychological stress—the death of a close relative, his uncle, to whom he was deeply attached. Because his emotional reactions were closely associated with his physical symptoms, he was treated both medically and psychiatrically. The collaboration of the surgical, medical, and psychiatry services of the Massachusetts General Hospital was responsible for the patient's ultimate improvement.

In addition to his ulcerative colitis, the patient had so many character defects, such a variety of emotional problems, and such a complexity of psychological symptoms that it is almost meaningless to attempt to classify him under a psychiatric diagnosis. According to Stanley Cobb, psychosomatic medicine in general is "that field of medicine in which the psychiatrist and the internist can advantageously work together in the study and treatment of disease."[1] Cobb lists nine groups of diseases that might be considered as fulfilling the above criterion, and ulcerative colitis is one of them.

There has been criticism of the term "psychosomatic" because of the implied dichotomy between the words psychological and somatic. This dichotomy should not exist. Every illness has its emotional components, but in certain illnesses, where there is a preponderance of psychological factors, some investigators have been led to consider the possibility of a causal relationship between a psychological

[1] H. W. Miles, S. Cobb, and H. Shands, *Case Histories in Psychosomatic Medicine* (New York: W. W. Norton, 1952).

trauma and the onset of the medical disease. Ulcerative colitis is such a disorder. In this study I shall not attempt to review the whole voluminous literature on the disease. I would, however, like to emphasize the salient points of some of the important papers dealing with this subject.

Since Cecil D. Murray has emphasized the importance of psychogenic factors in ulcerative colitis,[2] there is a general consensus that some patients have emotional difficulties and deal with them by inadequate psychological mechanisms. In some of the cases that have been studied psychiatrically, the onset of ulcerative colitis was frequently related to emotional stress. Erich Lindemann, who has studied extensively the psychological aspects of the treatment of such patients, has found that the patient depends on a key figure in his own environment for emotional security.[3] The loss of such a person (not only through death, but also through rejection, disillusionment, mental illness, or physical illness leading to the temporary incapacitation of that obligating partner) usually precedes the onset of the ulcerative colitis. He emphasized that, following this loss, the patient's mental state during the acute phase of the disease may often be that of a morbid grief reaction. Psychotic manifestations in patients with ulcerative colitis are also likely to be encountered, particularly if the psychiatrist explores deeply the patient's sexual adjustment. Such an exploration has a tendency to give rise to paranoid and severely morbid grief reactions or to somatic delusions similar to those encountered in individuals suffering from involutional depression, thus producing a marked deterioration of the patient's psychological adjustment.

[2] C. D. Murray, "Psychogenic Factors in the Etiology of Ulcerative Colitis and Bloody Diarrhea," *American Journal of Medical Science*, 180:239 (1930).

[3] E. Lindemann, "Modifications in the Course of Ulcerative Colitis in Relationship to Changes in Life Situations and Reactions Patterns," from Association for Research in Nervous and Mental Disease, *Life Stress and Bodily Disease*, 29:706–723 (1950).

In his paper "Ulcerative Colitis," Louis Zetzel also discusses the effect of psychogenic factors in the functioning of the colon.[4] He reports that there is agreement about the influence of such factors on functional changes of the colon, but adds that there is no proof that such disturbances can of themselves give rise to the inflammation and ulceration that are characteristic of ulcerative colitis. He concludes that immaturity and dependency are prominent personality characteristics.

Grace, Wolf, and Wolf in their book, *The Human Colon*, studied in detail nineteen patients with ulcerative colitis.[5] The patients were outwardly calm and placid but behind this façade were found to be intensely hostile, resentful, and guilty. These feelings, in addition, were associated with hyperfunction of the colon, increased motility, vascularity, fragility of the mucous membranes, and increased amounts of lysozyme. The authors concluded that the human colon is likely to react to threatening life situations and interpersonal problems. Change involving colonic hyperfunction when sustained may result in structural damage and disease. A constructive doctor-patient relationship plays an important part in obtaining favorable therapeutic results.

The bowel may act as a spokesman for sexual and aggressive attitudes, and the interruption of a dependent relationship can be followed rapidly by bloody diarrhea. The symptoms of ulcerative colitis appear to be a concomitant of the associated emotional conflict—according to John Nemiah.[6]

Various authors who have studied the psychological problems encountered in ulcerative colitis have in one way or

---

[4] L. Zetzel, "Ulcerative Colitis," *New England Journal of Medicine*, 251.15–16:601–615, 653–658 (1954).
[5] W. I. Grace, S. Wolf, and H. G. Wolf, *The Human Colon* (New York: Paul B. Hoeber, 1951).
[6] H. Lief, V. Lief, and N. Lief, *The Psychological Basis of Medical Practice* (New York: Paul B. Hoeber, 1963).

another emphasized early dependent needs. In his paper "Studies of Ulcerative Colitis," G. L. Engel, from psychologic data of thirty-nine patients with ulcerative colitis, observes that there is a characteristic type of dependent and restricted relationship with people.[7] He emphasized the significance of the mother-child symbiosis in determining the particular character of these patients and their vulnerability to separation, and believes that the disease develops only in the presence of such effects as helplessness, hopelessness, and despair. In addition, the emotions of fear, rage, and anxiety were mentioned by other authors. It is possible that such effects, coupled with a strong dependency, immaturity, and a need for a symbiotic relationship, point to very early mother-infant interaction and the possible traumatic situations that are likely to arise from it.

G. E. Daniels and his team of psychiatrists and gastroenterologists, reviewing thirty years of observation and treatment of ulcerative colitis, describe an intensive follow-up study of fifty-seven patients who had definite ulcerative colitis and received psychotherapy.[8] Having developed physical and psychological rating scales, they reviewed their findings systematically and found that a serious psychiatric diagnosis, such as schizophrenia, was a reliable and poor prognostic variable of the patient's physical and mental status. A good psychotherapeutic relationship seemed in general to have a beneficial effect on the patient's life adjustment, career, marriage, and family.

The psychotherapeutic approach for this kind of psychological disturbance requires a long supportive contact. This implies that an attempt should be made on the part of the

[7] G. L. Engel, "Studies of Ulcerative Colitis," *American Journal of Medicine*, 19:231–256 (August 1955).
[8] G. E. Daniels, J. F. O'Connor, A. Karush, L. Moses, C. A. Flood, and M. Lepore, "Three Decades in the Observation and Treatment of Ulcerative Colitis," *Psychosomatic Medicine*, 24:85–93 (1962).

therapist to help the patient deal with reality, for it is in this area that the patient's inadequate character encounters repeated failures. In such a treatment situation, the psychiatrist "lends himself" to the patient in order to help him to achieve a successful way of handling the emotional crises in his everyday life.

Although dependence is stressed in many psychiatric reviews of the psychological factors in ulcerative colitis, it appears that the degree or depth of the dependent needs varies considerably. One must raise the question of what is meant exactly by the word "dependence." Is it the dependence of the infant upon his mother, or is it the dependence of an adult upon his therapist? Can one equate the two, as has commonly been done? The story that follows is an attempt to present a picture of an "anaclitic type of relationship." [9]

The term "anaclitic" was first introduced by Freud in his paper "On Narcissism." It literally means "leaning on type," and it has to do with the child's attachment to his mother, or her substitute, for satisfaction of his nutritional needs. I have used the term here to describe the relationship of an adult patient who was helped to depend totally upon his therapist.[10] My observations on this relationship and its effects upon the patient are presented in detail in the following chapters.

[9] S. Freud, *The Complete Psychological Works of Sigmund Freud* (London: Hogarth Press, 1957), XIV, 87.
[10] A résumé has appeared in "Anaclitic Treatment in a Patient with Ulcerative Colitis," S. Cobb, ed., *American Journal of Medicine*, 14:731–735 (June 1953).

CHAPTER I

THE PATIENT

TOM WAS born in New York in 1910. His mother always considered him a problem, according to the stories his grandmother told him and occasional sarcastic comments from his mother. She had tried to breast-feed him on several occasions, although she had never wanted to; but he nursed so voraciously, apparently, that she gave it up in disgust and switched to a formula, which promptly gave the infant diarrhea. This feeding problem and the attacks of diarrhea continued throughout the first three years of his life. At times the diarrhea was so severe as to require a doctor's treatment, which angered the mother because so much money had to be spent on medical bills. This gave his mother another reason for disliking the boy, since she was a compulsively clean woman and hated to change diapers. She thought that his gastrointestinal difficulties were caused by his eating too much of the foods she disapproved of. He remembered that once his mother threw away a whole new box of candy and refused to return it to him despite his pleadings.

When Tom was three years old, his father died. He had been sick with cancer of the lung for some time, and Tom remembered his coughing and spitting blood. When Tom was three and a half years old, he went to live with his grandmother, and the next six years of his life were essentially happy ones. His grandmother was a maternal type of woman and apparently showered him with a great deal of affection, in contrast with his mother, whom Tom described as a cold individual, with a biting tongue, a horrible temper, and "snakelike" qualities. He was terrified of his mother. During this time his brother, who was four years older than Tom, lived with the mother one block away from where Tom lived. He said that, although his mother disliked him, she loved his brother. Tom did not remember any visit from his mother during the six years he lived with his grandmother. He did remember his grandmother telling him that his mother had remarried when he was eight years old, but they never came to visit Tom.

On one occasion, a year later, Tom's paternal uncle came to visit his grandmother. This was his introduction to a man who would exert a great influence upon his life. Tom felt immediately that his uncle disliked him very much. He talked a good deal about Tom's brother and about how happy he was not to have to take care of a "dirty brat" like Tom. The grandmother defended him, saying that he behaved very well and that his work at school was above reproach. She said she was shocked by his mother's and stepfather's attitude toward the boy. The uncle defended them and answered in a derogatory manner, saying that he was indifferent about good grades and wished that Tom were a little girl because he liked to play with little girls and fondle them. Tom remembered this visit very vividly. The next time he saw his uncle was at his grandmother's funeral, about two years later, when he was nine years old.

His grandmother died suddenly of a heart attack, and Tom talked about her death as being the biggest blow of his life. He had awakened early that morning and had got himself dressed and ready for school. Usually his grandmother would be preparing his breakfast at this time, but that day when he went down to the kitchen there was no breakfast. Wondering what could have happened, he went up to his grandmother's room and found her gasping for breath.

Foamy material was coming out of her mouth, and horrible sounds were audible from her chest. The thought came to his mind that she was "drowning in a sea of bubbles," and he could not understand how this could have happened. He rushed to her bedside and tried to get her to talk. She made a feeble attempt to communicate with him but was unable to do so. He then ran to a neighbor's house for help—screaming, shouting, crying, pleading. By the time help arrived, his grandmother was already dead.

When his mother, stepfather, and brother came to the house to see his grandmother, Tom wanted to run away from them. During the funeral Tom showed no emotion. He stared at his grandmother's face as she lay inside the coffin, but could not believe she was dead. He thought she was asleep and would wake up at any moment and speak to him. He thought over and over, "All is black; there is nothing." At the cemetery, he remembered staring down into the grave. "It was like a black hole," he said. He had an almost irresistible urge to jump into it and be with his grandmother forever.

From this time on, life was a nightmare for Tom. He had to live with his paternal uncle, his wife, and their daughter, and he received innumerable beatings here. One of the things that terrified him was that his aunt would not cut his hair, insisting that it be allowed to grow so it would look like her daughter's. He was teased unmercifully at school because of this, but whenever he asked his aunt to cut his hair she would give him a beating. This was usually followed by another beating from his uncle, who said he had wanted Tom to be a girl. On one occasion he tried to cut his own hair, but the attempt resulted in his having short hair on one side of his head and long curls on the other. He was the laughing stock of the school for many weeks.

Tom's descriptions of these various episodes were always

given with much feeling. Although it was difficult to determine how much was fantasy and how much was reality, still it was apparent that he had a great deal of emotional investment in these childhood experiences.

Tom could recall very little more about his life with his uncle and aunt for the next four years. The uncle had a vegetable garden, and Tom remembered that he was required to do hard manual work in the garden after school and on weekends, but he was able to perform these tasks very well and consequently earned considerable amounts of money for his uncle. Because of this, the uncle and his wife soon gave up their efforts to make him look like a girl and encouraged him to work harder to earn more money for them. He continued to do good work at school and repeatedly made the honor roll.

One day when he was thirteen years old, a "monumental" event occurred in his relationship with his uncle. He had worked hard all day in the garden and had then gone to the market and sold all the produce at a good price. When he returned home, his uncle called him to the cellar and asked him for the money. When Tom showed him the amount he had secured, his uncle could not believe his eyes. He seemed to be particularly pleased. The uncle had been drinking throughout the day and was in a somewhat drunken condition. As a sign of appreciation for the boy's hard work, he offered Tom a drink. One drink followed another, and soon they were both intoxicated. Tom remembered this episode as a turning point in his life. It was the beginning of a very friendly relationship with his uncle, whose attitude toward Tom changed completely. From bitter hatred, he developed a strong attachment for Tom and on many occasions took Tom's side in arguments with his wife. Tom worked for his uncle throughout his teens, and after graduating from high school continued to earn a great deal of money for him. During all this time Tom had no outside friends, either boys or girls. His uncle was the center of his life and their drinking together in the cellar his only fun.

At the age of twenty-one, Tom, following one of the drinking episodes with his uncle, met the daughter of a next-door neighbor in the street. He asked her to come down to the cellar for a drink and she accepted immediately. She was older than Tom, in both years and experience, and with no difficulty seduced him into having intercourse with her. Soon after this she announced to him her pregnancy and her expectation of marriage. Tom agreed without realizing what he was getting himself into. Soon after, she denied the whole thing and married another man. Tom felt hurt by her behavior and, in recounting all of this, said that he felt like a little boy who was told what to do and obediently did it. His mother's temper, his fear of his aunt, and the unpredictable behavior of his first girlfriend were constantly on his mind. He did, however, meet another girl whom he decided to marry; on his wedding day he became so upset that he thought of running away. His wife soon became pregnant. Tom was apprehensive about becoming a father, but he also felt very proud. His uncle reassured him and jokingly added that maybe the expected baby would be a girl—something he himself had wished for all of his life.

In the next nine years Tom's wife presented him with four boys. He pictured his wife as powerful, able to care for and discipline the children, and in full control of the household. She was somewhat extravagant, but Tom was unable to stop her spending or prevent her from doing what she pleased. He said, "A weakness or a paralysis would come on me and I would freeze, having nothing to say to her." Yet he continued to work hard and earn a good deal of money, and he could not understand why he was so weak and incapable of running his own family. He said, frowning, that he felt just as he did when he was a little boy and was unable to cope with his aunt's overpowering strength. Even though he realized that his wife was not as strong as he pictured her, he felt unable to do anything about it. Most of the money he made was carelessly spent; his family lived in poverty.

When Tom was twenty-nine years old he left his family. Despite threats from the church and neighbors, as well as from social agencies and the police, he did not return. He established a close relationship with an old woman who was living with her granddaughter, a girl to whom Tom was closely attached. He went into hiding in her house. Tom also developed a closer relationship with his first-born son, who, by that time, was eleven years old. The boy would come to meet his father, and quite often Tom would offer him a drink, as his uncle had done with him. He had one or two friends whom he described as social outcasts.

In spite of the difficulties he was encountering during that time, Tom claims that he was happy. He actually enjoyed being followed and threatened by social workers and priests. He described one occasion when he had a long discussion with a priest about his "moral life." It gave him "great delight" to be able to argue and hold his own against the better-educated priest, and to finally convince him that there were strong psychological reasons why he was compelled to behave the way he did. He described his relationship with the old woman as a happy one. She always had a lavish meal ready for him when he came back from his work. She was thrifty with the money he gave her, and always affectionate and loving. She treated him like a child, and he often thought of his grandmother when he was with her. She was so much older than he was that he felt protected by her. There was never any question of sex. She provided him with a warmth he had not experienced since his grandmother's death. Tom did a considerable amount of drinking during this time, but he was always able to go to his job the next morning and to work hard.

Quite frequently Tom visited his uncle, who by then had separated from his wife and was living alone. They always had "wonderful times" together, going down to the cellar to drink or going to a local tavern, where Tom felt that everyone liked him and understood his troubles. He and his uncle would always reminisce about their first experience in drinking together. Tom said he felt that he had under-estimated his uncle when he was a child. He thought the man had been the victim of his aunt's temper, even more than he himself had been, and that the efforts to make Tom look like a girl were the wish of his aunt much more than of his uncle. He also felt that the beatings his uncle had given him were usually associated with the uncle's rage against his wife and an inability to express his angry feelings toward her, and that Tom had been used as a scapegoat. This psychological explanation and rationalization seemed to make him very happy.

During these visits with his uncle, Tom would find him-self thinking of his own father and remembering him as a kindly person who would "never harm a fly." He recalled that his father, on one occasion before his illness, had told him the story of his life. The only thing he could remember well was his father's love for machines and how fascinated he was when his father had taken a toy car apart and put it back together again. He had kept this car and had given it to his oldest son. He also remembered his father's being sick and spitting up blood. This thought was always associated with his father's death, and it would bring to mind the death of his grandmother in somewhat similar circumstances. In contrast with these pleasant, even though sad, thoughts, his memories about his aunt were always unpleasant. His mother's domineering and "snappy" ways, her terrible temper, and her "snakelike coldness" would also come back to him, and he would become paralyzed with fear. It was then that he would take two or three glasses of beer or wine to forget. His animosity against his wife was not so pronounced.

One Sunday afternoon, when Tom was thirty-one years old, he went to visit his uncle. It was a beautiful summer day, and they were both sitting in the garden and drinking. Tom was deep in thought when he suddenly noticed his uncle clutching his chest, making peculiar sounds in his attempt to breathe, and unable to move. Tom suddenly felt paralyzed. He saw his uncle gasping for breath and moaning with pain, but in Tom's mind there was only one thought: "He is dying like my grandmother." He was unable to speak or even raise his hand to help his uncle in any way. The uncle's agony did not last long; he was dead in a few minutes.

The neighbors, who had heard the moans, came rushing in and found Tom staring blankly at the lifeless body. He did not know how long he remained in that position, but after a while two people shook him and told him he needed a rest. All that night he walked aimlessly through the streets, and finally, early in the morning, he arrived at his old friend's home, where he collapsed in bed. Later that day, Tom woke up from his deep sleep with severe abdominal cramps and an equally severe attack of diarrhea, such as he had not experienced since his early childhood. Further attacks of diarrhea, with bloody bowel movements, occurred quite often during the next few months. Finally, weak and exhausted, he decided to come to the emergency ward of the hospital. He was admitted for a diagnosis of his medical problems, and a report of acute ulcerative colitis was made.

Before going further, an attempt should be made to evaluate the patient's personality, keeping in mind his past history.

One is impressed by the three serious losses that Tom experienced in his life: his father, his grandmother, and his uncle. He lost the people whom he had learned to like and for whom he had warm feelings that were reciprocated by them. In contrast, any such relationship with his mother, whom he described as "strong and domineering," was nonexistent; his feelings toward her and for his aunt were invariably colored by strong fear, at times verging on panic, that paralyzed him and made him unable to cope with them. Interestingly enough, he showed this same reaction to his wife. Although outwardly she appeared to be different from his mother, still Tom felt unable to deal with her and her financial extravagances, despite the fact that he earned a good living. This inability to deal with his wife stemmed from the same paralyzing fears he had experienced with his mother, and he finally had to flee.

Tom was an intelligent man, well liked, and a hard worker. Outwardly, he appeared to be close to people. They thought of him as being very amusing and original. Inwardly, however, he was afraid of people and never really trusted anyone emotionally. With his old woman friend, he attempted to relive his experience with his grandmother, which had been the only happy time of his life. In the same way, he attempted to establish a relationship with his oldest son similar to the one he had established with his uncle. It is of interest that, during the drinking bouts with the uncle, he remembered and pondered his early experiences with his father.

In sum: Tom had a limited number of close relationships, all of them ending with deaths. He was industrious, intelligent, and hard-working; but in his other interpersonal relations he was distant and frightened almost to the point of being incapable of functioning, despite the fact that he made a good outward appearance and was liked by others.

CHAPTER II

THE MEDICAL PROBLEM

TOM WAS admitted to the Massachusetts General Hospital for the first time, complaining of recurring attacks of diarrhea of six months' duration. This illness began approximately six months before an admission to another hospital for an upper respiratory infection. Tom had said at that time that he "took a cold" during exposure to unusually severe wet wintry weather. The cold was characterized by a sore throat and nasal discharge, and it was then, for the first time, that Tom had mentioned an intermittent colic epigastric pain with the diarrhea. This condition had lasted for two weeks. It was learned subsequently from the patient that this attack of cold and diarrhea had followed closely upon his uncle's death.

In the six months before his first admission, Tom had five or six similar attacks, each one lasting for one or two weeks. During these periods he usually had eight to ten bowel movements a day. The stools were loose and accompanied by a great deal of gas. The character of his stools had not been constant: sometimes they were almost entirely of clear fluid, and on other occasions he had detected undigested particles of food or pieces of skinlike material. He had also noticed blood in his stools a few times, but this had not been the general rule. He did not mention the presence of any mucus in the stools.

During the first attack of diarrhea he had vomited a great deal, but this had not been repeated. There had been no blood in his vomitus. He had frequently had mild chills during these attacks, but the chills were never accompanied by shivering. He had experienced only what he described as chilly sensations all over his body. He did not know whether he had had a fever or not, but said he was usually hot and that he had perspired a great deal. The pain during the early attacks was localized in a small area above the umbilicus, in the middle line, and it was found upon palpation that this region was tender. More recently, however, the pain had descended to below the umbilicus. There had been no constant relationship between his food and his physical condition, but Tom had the impression that his food was responsible for these occasional attacks.

He had never quite recovered from the upper respiratory infection that preceded his gastrointestinal disturbance. He had had a moderate cough, productive of a thick mucoid substance, ever since that time, and he claimed that this type of cough had developed for the first time during the preceding winter. His nose had discharged mucus throughout this period. Four months before admission, he had noticed for the first time a feeling of tightness across his lower chest whenever he took a deep breath. This he described as not a real pain, but rather as a feeling that his chest expansion was limited. At that time he consulted his local doctor, who X-rayed Tom's chest, made a diagnosis of "influenza pleurisy, intestinal flu, and chronic sore throat," and sent him briefly to another hospital. He said the X-ray showed no evidence of tuberculosis. During the past two months Tom said he had occasionally coughed up a blood-tinged sputum, but that he had never had a frank hemoptysis. Also during this time he had experienced fatigue and noticed that he perspired freely on exertion. He claimed he had maintained his usual rugged appetite throughout the illness, and he did not believe he had lost much weight.

Family history. The father died of cancer when Tom

was only three years old, and his mother had married again, as mentioned already. She was now sixty-three years old and was said not to be in good health, having recently lost a great deal of weight. Tom had one older brother and several half-brothers and half-sisters. There was no diabetes or hypertension in the family. (The social history will be omitted here since it will be discussed in detail in the next chapter.)

Past medical history. Tom's general health had been reasonably good prior to the onset of the present illness. He had had chicken pox, mumps, and whooping cough as a child, and was also thought to have had chronic bronchitis as an adolescent. He had had three previous hospitalizations—one for tonsillectomy at the age of three years, another for removal of the semilunar cartilage following an injury to his knee while he was working at a lumber mill two years before the present admission, and the one already mentioned.

System review. Tom claimed that, approximately six weeks before, "red blotches" had appeared on his skin, particularly on his face and arms. This rash would disappear within an hour's time and was not associated with his food. He also said he had had pains and aches for the past eight years, particularly in his elbows and knees. He had been told that he had arthritis, but the pains had not interfered with his work. One month prior to admission, he noticed that the cervical glands were swollen, but he had been told that this was associated with his sore throat. There had been attacks of headache on several occasions and a feeling of pressure in his head that was associated with anxiety about his physical condition; but he remembered that, as a child, he had severe headaches and that at times these headaches were accompanied by "blind spots" in the field of his vision and by a numbness of his eyes. He had always been farsighted and had been troubled by astigmatism. He complained of double vision when he looked at objects within a distance of two or three feet. He said his eyelids had been red and swollen for a long time, and he had frequently noticed pus in his eyes. He had a chronically runny nose, particularly in cold weather. Cardiovascular system review disclosed that Tom had been told that he had hypertension when he was young, and during the past eight years he had experienced palpitations of the heart, five or six times. Tom had always had an abnormally large appetite. His teeth were in very bad condition. Before the onset of his present illness, he had not had difficulty with his gastrointestinal system, except for hemorrhoidal trouble. He complained of occasional urgency on urination and, at times, of being incontinent of urine, but this was always associated with drinking too much. The review of the central nervous system was essentially negative.

In sum: A man thirty-one years of age entered the hospital with recurrent attacks of diarrhea and abdominal pain of six months' duration. He had noted blood in his stools several times. On one occasion these attacks were accompanied by vomiting. During the six months before admission, the patient had a chronic respiratory infection and had noticed easy fatigue.

On physical examination there was evidence of acneform eruption over his face, shoulders, and chest. There was a dry discharge in both eyes, partially congested turbinates with considerable exudate on the right side, carious teeth, large and small lymph nodes, and tenderness in the inguinal and axillary regions. The blood pressure was 148 over 104. The heart was essentially negative and the lung fields were clear. There was diffuse tenderness over the abdomen, particularly pronounced at the left lower quadrant, and the presence of two small, soft penile ulcers. The diagnosis was early ulcerative colitis and essential hypertension.

The laboratory tests were as follows: Fasting blood sugar was 82 mg. percent, nonprotein nitrogen was 29 mg. percent, and the total protein was 6.5 gm. Three urine analyses were negative. The blood count was normal. Stool examination showed no evidence of amoebic cyst or other parasites.

The patient had a sigmoidoscopy that revealed a red granular mucosa, with a considerable amount of mucus. There were no bleeding points, but the wall was pink and guaiac positive. The bowel wall was cultured and showed evidence of a growing Staphylococcus albus. These findings were thought to be consistent with early ulcerative colitis. Another sigmoidoscopy, performed ten days later, showed evidence of red granular mucosa. There was moderate spasm, and the bowel bled easily. Several tiny pinpoint bleeding ulcerations were seen. The appearance of the bowel was consistent with the diagnosis of ulcerative colitis.

During his hospitalization, Tom was treated with sulfadiazine and penicillin. He showed slow but good progress. Extensive psychiatric evaluation was carried on throughout his hospital stay. He was discharged with a diagnosis of ulcerative colitis and was followed in the out-patient gastrointestinal clinic and the psychiatry clinic. His total hospital stay was two and a half months.

Three months later it became necessary for Tom to be readmitted to the hospital. His appetite had begun to fail, and moderate abdominal cramps had developed that usually lasted for over half an hour during each attack. These symptoms had become more pronounced in the two weeks prior to his second admission. During the five hours before he arrived at the hospital, Tom had about ten watery bowel movements and, in addition, a urinary frequency and urgency had developed. Physical examination revealed a robust and well-nourished man who was in no distress. He still showed poor dental hygiene. There was acneform eruption

on the anterior chest base and lower extremities. The heart
and lungs were normal. There was a slight epigastric and
lower-quadrant tenderness, with generalized lack of relaxa-
tion. Some hemorrhoidal tabs and slight sphincter spasm
were noted. The prostate was slightly enlarged and tender,
with no secretions expressed on massage. His white blood
count and hemoglobin were normal throughout his hospital
stay. Urine analyses were negative. Several stool examinations were guaiac positive. The total protein was 6.8 gm.
percent and the NPN was 34 mg. percent. The patient was
placed on bed rest, given a low-residue 3,500 calorie diet,
and was atropinized. He was seen on several occasions by
the psychiatrist who had been following him in the psychiatry clinic. On this regime he quieted down very rapidly.
There was one exacerbation of pain and diarrhea that lasted
a few hours, but otherwise he remained symptom-free for
several days and was soon allowed to go home. The diagnosis was exacerbation of chronic nonspecific ulcerative
colitis. This hospitalization had lasted for a period of three
weeks.

Three months later Tom again had a brief hospitalization.
He was admitted this time by the orthopedic service because
of a tenderness and pain that had developed in his left knee.
Soon after this admission, however, there was a flare-up of
his colitis, with several bowel movements a day. On one
occasion gross blood was noted in his stool. When he also
complained of moderate lower-abdominal cramps, he was
transferred from the orthopedic to the medical service. He
claimed that this attack of ulcerative colitis was precipitated
by an emotional upset. He was seen by the same therapist in
consultation from the psychiatry service. After the ulcerative colitis subsided, he was again transferred back to the
orthopedic service, where an excision of the medial meniscus
of his left knee joint was performed. Because the meniscus

was found to be torn, its removal was necessary. His post-operative recovery was uneventful, and he was soon discharged. Again he was followed by the psychiatry and orthopedic clinics, this time for the next eight months. During this time, Tom lost two of his toes in an accident at work. Following this, a mild exacerbation of his ulcerative colitis developed, with three to four stools per day. A week before another return to the hospital, the number of stools had increased to ten a day. On the day of his admission there were nineteen. These stools contained a great deal of mucus, but only small amounts of blood. There was also associated abdominal pain, particularly in the left lower quadrant. Tom had eaten sparsely during the three days before admission and had vomited on two occasions. When asked about his toes, he said he had lost them in an accident, and he blamed his psychiatrist for having recommended that he return to his job. During the physical examination the blood pressure was 135 over 100, and the pulse was 72. There were many small maculopapular lesions over the chest and back, and a pair of nodose lesions on the calf of the left leg. The heart was normal in size, the sounds of good quality. The lung fields were clear. The abdomen was tender to palpation throughout, but particularly in the left lower quadrant. The peristalsis was very active, and the prostate was one and a half times larger than normal. Neurological examination revealed hyperactive reflexes. The laboratory tests showed a six million red blood count and a hemoglobin of 16.5 gm. The white blood count was 11,000, with 81 percent polymorphonuclear cells, 4 percent large lymphocytes, 13 percent small lymphocytes, and 2 percent monocytes. The red blood cells and the platelets were normal. Urine analyses were negative and so were stool examinations for pathogens, but several stools were guaiac positive. The patient was placed on a low-residue diet of 3,000

calories with 150 gm. of protein. In addition, he was put on
bed rest and received 0.75 cc. tincture of opium every 6
hours and 100 mg. of seconal for sleep. He improved rapidly
on this regime, and two days prior to discharge he was
having only one solid stool daily. He had been seen by a
skin consultant, as well as his regular psychiatrist, throughout his hospital stay.

During the next three years Tom was followed in the
gastrointestinal, skin, and orthopedic clinics, and he made
occasional visits to the emergency ward, but these visits were
related to emotional upsets that sometimes followed his
regular interviews in the psychiatry clinic. He had a brief
admission to the hospital because of a perianal abscess,
which was incised and drained, and was followed subsequently by a few visits in the surgical clinic.

His fifth admission to the Massachusetts General Hospital
was after a seven-month interval following his short admission for treatment of the perianal abscess. During this time
Tom had done well, apparently, but in the last month a
mucoid drainage from the anal region had developed and
he complained of pain, for which he took paregoric in large
amounts. His diet was inadequate, and in the last few weeks
daily watery stools had developed again. There were occasional hemorrhages consisting of several ounces of bright
red blood which, he said, followed a sudden urge to def-
ecate. It was now that Tom admitted, for the first time,
that he had left his wife and was living with another woman.
He claimed that he had "the best deal" he had ever had,
because he received a great deal of help from this woman.

The physical examination on admission, besides the usual
findings that have been mentioned before, revealed a grey-
white shaggy fissure in the anterior wall of the rectum, involving the sphincter. The laboratory tests were negative.
An excision of the anal fissure was made, and a carbuncle

that was discovered was opened and drained. The sigmoidos-copy performed at this time showed an essentially normal bowel. The patient suffered considerable pain postopera-tively, but was discharged from the hospital after a week's stay. Two months later he was again admitted because of an-other attack of recurrent diarrhea, which involved six to seven watery bowel movements a day, with passage of bright red blood and clots, accompanied by crampy low-abdominal pain. These symptoms had become intensified two weeks prior to admission. The physical examination found virtually the same conditions as had the previous ones: acne over the face and shoulders, abdominal tenderness in the left lower quadrant, and a granular fissurectomy wound. Laboratory data revealed hemoglobin of 10 gm. and a white count of 7000. During this hospitalization Tom was given three barium enemas, and it was finally concluded that there was a localized area of ulcerative colitis in the descending colon. The patient was practically asymptomatic during this stay in the hospital, except for repeated episodes of de-pression, and because of this the psychiatry service was called in consultation. Since the psychiatrist who had been following Tom during the past four years had finished his service at Massachusetts General Hospital, a new psychia-trist was called into the picture. It was the latter's impres-sion that the patient should attempt to get in touch with his old therapist rather than to become involved with a new one. The decision was reached, therefore, to have the patient discharged and seen on an out-patient basis if he could not continue with his previous psychiatrist. He was discharged on a low-residue diet, tincture of belladonna was prescribed, and instructions were given that he was to be followed as usual in the gastrointestinal clinic. During his stay in the hospital, stool examinations were repeatedly guaiac negative.

But within a short time, Tom had to re-enter the hospital because of recurrent attacks of abdominal cramps and bloody diarrhea, which he claimed had occurred off and on after his last discharge. He described this diarrhea as somewhat watery, sometimes bloody, and always associated with extreme constant pain in the left lower quadrant and in the anal region. He said the pain occasionally was an intermittent, crampy, left-abdominal one, radiating upwards and downwards and occurring at unpredictable times. It seemed to be temporarily relieved somewhat by a bowel movement or by passing gas by rectum. He claimed that on other occasions he had noticed a burning, clawing, steady umbilical pain which was associated with nausea, but there was no vomiting connected with it. This pain usually lasted for three or four hours and was relieved by massaging the abdominal area. He said his appetite had not been very good and that he had lost weight for the first time—nine pounds in a period of about five weeks. During this hospitalization, the surgical service was asked to see the patient in consultation in order to decide what should be done with this man who had had several hospital admissions and who seemed to be growing progressively worse. After several discussions between the gastrointestinal and surgical services, it was decided that an operation was probably the next logical step, but it was felt that the psychiatry service should also be consulted.

A letter was written to Tom's previous psychiatrist, asking for his opinion regarding an operation. A meeting was arranged. The patient's psychiatric problem was discussed at length by three psychiatrists, and the decision was reached that there was no serious psychiatric contraindication to interfere with surgery. This was told to the patient, who promised to cooperate and so was transferred to the surgical service. He was transfused with 1,000 cc. of blood for two days, given sulfathalidine, and was operated upon. A sub-total colectomy was performed. The areas of disease involved the upper part of the ascending colon, the transverse, the lower part of the descending colon, and the major part of the sigmoid. The mucosa was ulcerated and presented granular and, in some places, dark red hemorrhagic discolorations. The lateral margins of these ulcerations were markedly edematous; the bases were dark red, granular, and in some places coated with a dirty grey-yellow, puslike substance. The serosa was injected and attached to the surrounding structures by a few fine adhesions.

Tom did well postoperatively. His hemoglobin was normal. A well-regulated ileostomy with a well-fitting ileostomy bag seemed to function adequately. There was a slight discharge from his rectum which had been left intact because it was found to be normal and a decision was reached to leave it as a "blind pouch" so that eventually the patient might have an anastomosis. Tom was discharged in good condition three weeks after the operation.

He again was followed in the psychiatry clinic, as well as in the surgical and gastrointestinal clinics; but very soon after he left the hospital, he went on a "seven-day binge," did not eat adequately, did not take care of his ileostomy bag, and drank a great amount of alcohol. During the next two months, his alcohol intake increased considerably and he started to deteriorate psychiatrically. He began to come for his psychiatric interviews in an intoxicated condition, until finally he developed auditory hallucinations and appeared to be seriously depressed. It was because of these symptoms that he was admitted to the psychiatry service for the first time.

The results of his physical examination on admission were essentially the same as during his previous hospitalizations. His blood pressure was 150 over 104. A grade I apical

systolic heart murmur was heard, and A-2 was louder than
P-2. The lung fields were clear. Abdominal examination
revealed a well-healed left rectal scar and an adequate-ap-
pearing ileostomy, except for a deep red edematous area
surrounding it. The surgical service was called in consultation for recommendations concerning his ileostomy care and
the areas of inflammation. In consultation, it was thought
that the ileostomy was functioning quite adequately and
that the patient's difficulties were primarily psychiatric. The
area of inflammation around the ileostomy was thought to
be due to neglect, associated with and following his alcoholic
indulgences. The patient's course in the psychiatry ward
will be discussed in detail in the next chapter.

Tom was visited by his first psychiatrist and, after a
period of about a month and a half, his psychiatric symptoms improved greatly and he was transferred from the
closed to the open psychiatry ward. But as he improved
psychiatrically, blood and mucus started to leak from his
rectum. Since this discharge increased progressively, the
thought was entertained that ulcerations had developed in
the area of the rectum that was left intact at the time of his
original colectomy. In view of this, another surgical consultation was held to discuss the best procedure to follow.
The surgeons agreed that the patient probably had ulcerative
colitis and recommended total removal of the rectum; but,
in a subsequent consultation, the surgeons reversed their
opinions, feeling that not only would resection of the patient's rectum be a sizeable procedure, involving some risk
to the patient, but they felt that such a procedure could not
be justified on the basis of only a slight discharge from the
rectum. They said that if the patient were to develop severe
rectal bleeding, the possibility of surgery might again be
considered. In a subsequent note, two days later, the surgeons reverted to their original conviction that the rectal

discharge of blood, pus, and mucus was convincing evidence of ulcerations of the rectum, and that an operation was indicated. When it was definitely decided that the patient should be operated upon, he was transferred to the surgical service, and soon after had a combined abdominal perineal resection of part of the sigmoid and rectum.

The pathology report revealed that a segment of the sigmoid and the rectum, including the anus and measuring 21 cm., had been removed. The wall was slightly thickened. The mucosa was generally reddened and slightly granular, but retained fairly normal folds. At 1.5 cm. from the proximal resection edge there was a deep fold of normal-appearing mucosa that extended completely around the circumference of the sigmoid and was raised 1 cm. from the mucosa surface. Immediately distal to this was an irregular stellate, poorly circumscribed, ulcerated area measuring 3 mm. by 5 mm. and containing dark red clotted blood in its space. No other ulcers were noticed. The exposed serosal surface was smooth and glistening. Many reddish-tan succulent lymph nodes—the largest measuring 1 cm.—were present in the surrounding fat. The patient did well postoperatively, but required narcotics for control of pain. It was thought that more psychotherapy was necessary, and so he was again transferred to the psychiatry ward.

One month after the operation, it was found that the patient's operative wound was closing very satisfactorily. There was relatively little discomfort from the drainage, and he was given instructions in the care of his ileostomy. The additional medical problems involving this patient will be discussed in subsequent chapters, because they are intimately related to his psychiatric problems.

CHAPTER III

THE PSYCHIATRIC PROBLEM

TOM'S emotional reactions at the onset of his medical illness have been described in the previous chapter. It was because these emotional difficulties were recognized early by the medical staff that he was referred to the psychiatry service for consultation and then was taken over as a psychiatric patient, assigned a psychiatrist for therapy, and followed in the psychiatry clinic for four years. During this period he was admitted to the hospital on several occasions because of exacerbations of his ulcerative colitis, or for such complications as perineal abscesses. Very little is known about what transpired in the out-patient psychiatry clinic during this particular phase of his psychiatric treatment, except that an attempt was made throughout the four years to give him the support that would help him to function independently on the outside, despite his medical complications. Generally speaking, he seemed to manage very well.

Toward the end of this four-year period, in the month of October, another exacerbation of his ulcerative colitis developed, and he was again admitted to the hospital, where he was treated with a conservative medical regime, while continuing to be seen by the psychiatry service. The deterioration in his physical condition at this time, however, was connected with the loss of his psychiatrist, who had finished his training and had decided to become associated with another hospital in the Boston area and to start his own private practice. This psychiatrist had discussed at length with Tom the possibility of his coming under the care of a new resident in the psychiatry clinic. Tom had at first expressed considerable anger about such a plan, but finally he agreed that this seemed to be the only solution. It was following his doctor's departure that he developed the exacerbation of his ulcerative colitis that led to his readmission to the hospital in October. He remained hospitalized for only a short time, however. He met his new psychiatrist and talked to him about his reactions to the loss of his previous therapist. He was favorably impressed by his new doctor and was amazed at his thorough familiarity with the problems. Arrangements were made for Tom's follow-up in the psychiatry clinic on a two-interviews-a-week basis.

During the next two months the medical symptoms continued to persist, and in December surgical intervention was considered for the first time. The patient was evaluated surgically; it was decided that his condition had become chronic and that an operation was necessary; and he was therefore admitted for a colectomy, as mentioned in the last chapter. He was operated upon and remained in the hospital for about three weeks.

His surgical recovery was uneventful. He gained weight and felt well. He was again discharged to the psychiatry clinic in the care of his therapist, but almost immediately alarming psychiatric symptoms began to appear. For the first time he became depressed, and this depression deepened despite the efforts of his psychotherapist to help him. He was seen three times a week in the clinic, but he still failed to respond. Hallucinations developed, and, in an attempt to silence the accusatory voices that became progressively more disturbing to him, he turned to alcohol. He drank heavily. The auditory hallucinations that he tried to "drown with whiskey" were urging him to kill everybody who was in authority, in general, and his previous psychiatrist, in particular. He recalled an incident that occurred one time when he was working on a construction job high on a bridge. He said that he suddenly felt a tremendous urge to smash the head of another worker with a heavy metal rod he was holding. When he realized what had happened, he became terrified that he had come so close to hitting the man. He said he felt paralyzed and had to be brought down forcibly by three other men because he was unable to move. On several occasions in the past, his auditory hallucinations took on a self-accusatory tone and urged him to commit suicide. Two or three times he caught himself standing on a bridge, looking down at the Mystic River, thinking of jumping and ending all his suffering. At another time he had the impulse to jump under the heavy tires of a big truck, hoping he would be smashed to death.

As the voices now increased in frequency, so did his consumption of alcohol. The only place where he felt secure was in the psychiatry clinic. He appeared to be relieved for a short time after each interview with his therapist, but soon the voices would come back. During his interviews he would lash out at his previous therapist, accusing him of abandoning him, as everybody else had abandoned him all through his life. The loss of the man who had done so much for him in the previous four years seemed to be something he could not cope with. He was angry most of the time, but at other times he seemed depressed. Yet he refused hospitalization on the psychiatry ward.

The next winter was a very stormy one for Tom. Many times he came to the emergency ward feeling that he was on the verge of killing himself or someone else. On one occasion, he found himself with a knife in his pocket, at the new office of his ex-psychiatrist, hoping the doctor would come out so that he could attack him. His depression grew steadily worse, and at times he was almost uncommunicative during his interviews. The homicidal ideas seemed to subside somewhat as the winter progressed, but when this happened the suicidal thoughts became progressively stronger. Finally, during one interview Tom admitted that he was afraid he would commit suicide, and he agreed with his doctor to be admitted to the hospital. This was in April, and it was his first admission for psychiatric reasons.

The main features of his mental status on this admission were profound depression, with some degree of motor agitation and suicidal ideas; marked tremulousness; fragmented stream of thought; preoccupation with threatening auditory hallucinations, at which time he would interrupt his conversation with the doctor in order to answer the threatening voices. In responding to these voices he assumed a trancelike facial expression. This was particularly noticeable when the voices urged him to kill members of his own family. His judgment and insight were poor, but an intact memory and orientation were noted. A physical examination revealed a muscular man with scattered pustular acneform rash on his face, and with rubbery clavicle and inguinal nodes that were easily palpable. The heart sounds were muffled. A grade I apical systolic murmur was audible. A-2 was louder than P-2. The blood pressure was 150 over 104. The lung fields were clear. An old left rectus scar that had healed well was visible. There was a well-functioning ileostomy that was surrounded by a deep red area with a pustular eruption, and several septic foci that were discharging serosanguineous material around the anal region. A neurological examination revealed no abnormalities. Laboratory tests showed a hemoglobin of eleven grams with an eight thousand white blood cell count. The urine was negative. A blood smear showed 81 percent polymorphonuclear cells and the rest lymphocytes. The red blood cells were hypochromic.

Tom was placed in the closed section of the psychiatry ward and was visited there daily by his resident psychiatrist. At first he remained profoundly depressed and continued to be frightened by the auditory hallucinations, but before long he began to show a marked improvement. His hallucinations decreased and soon disappeared. His depression also was less noticeable. Because of all this, Tom was quickly moved from the closed to the open ward, and soon he appeared to be asymptomatic emotionally, for the most part. On the other hand, his physical condition started to deteriorate. The pustular eruption in his abdomen became worse. The rectal discharge from the blind pouch of his rectum, which remained after his first operation, became increasingly bloody. On consultation with the surgical service it was decided that another operation was required for the total removal of the sigmoid and rectum, and Tom was again taken to the surgical service. This was in May.

The night before the operation Tom heard that his surgeon might not be on hand the next morning and that another doctor would have to replace him. He became very angry at this, and the resentment he had expressed against his previous psychiatrist who had left him was revived. He paced the floor, demanded to see his present psychiatrist immediately, and declared that he would not go through with the operation. He was easily quieted down, however, when he was told that all this was a false alarm and that he was going to be operated on by the doctor of his own choice.

The operation consisted of a combined abdominal perineal resection of the sigmoid and the rectum, under general anesthesia. Again his recovery was essentially uneventful, and he returned to the psychiatry service two weeks after surgery. The pathology report of the removed specimen of the sigmoid and rectum showed a slightly thickened wall with a reddened granular mucosa. A poorly circumscribed area of ulceration, 3 by 5 mm. and containing clotted blood at its base, was discovered in the distal area of the sigmoid. There were also many enlarged lymph nodes present in the surrounding fat. The diagnosis was "chronic ulcerative colitis."

In his psychotherapy, Tom talked about his past "rage reactions" following his first operation. He apparently had not discussed them with his therapist then, fearing that the new doctor would disapprove of him. Actually, it seems that these rage reactions preceded his depression at that time, which was followed by the auditory hallucinations, alcoholism, homicidal and suicidal ideas, and admission to the hospital. He denied feeling angry when these symptoms appeared, but he seemed to be deeply preoccupied with such thoughts before the second operation. He said that, although he realized that the discharge from his rectum was a threat to his very survival, he still at times wished he had not been operated upon again. On other occasions, however, he thought that the operation prevented his "cracking up." He also worried a great deal about his children, fearing they would make fun of him because he had no rectum.

In spite of these worries, Tom was quite active on the ward. He was outwardly friendly with many of the patients. He went to a ward party that was arranged in his honor as a "welcome back" by the other patients, and he seemed to enjoy the affair very much. A few days later he got permission to go home and visit his family. When he returned to the hospital he appeared to be in good spirits. He said that visiting his boys reminded him of his visits with his uncle when both of them got drunk.

In his subsequent interviews he again reminisced about his feelings before the second operation. He said that during the three days before surgery he was preoccupied with the fear that the surgeon who was going to operate on him—

whom he knew well, trusted, and liked—might make a mistake and kill him. This thought had worried him a great deal. He also talked about his hallucinations, which had completely disappeared, and said that when the voices started to recede he heard only "little whiny ones," and he remembered that one of these voices had told him that he should kill "little Tom." "Little Tom is not yet dead," the voice said, "but he must die." This seemed to have happened repeatedly, and he interpreted it as meaning that the surgery was going to fail and that he would die. It was then, he said, that he knew he was on the verge of insanity, and, despite his fear of the operation, he felt that it might perform a miracle and make him sane. He said that the insanity convictions came from resentment and fear, particularly from the feeling that others wanted to take advantage of him. But he said he had discovered there was also another part of him and this part tried to control everybody, to push them around, and at times it seemed that the best way to control them was to get rid of them once and for all. This thought terrified him, but he continued to talk about wanting to push people around—particularly people who were giving him a hard time.

Two weeks after his operation Tom developed pain in his back, owing to a urinary infection. He had already been placed on demerol postoperatively for pain, and this new complication triggered off a great deal of anxiety because he thought this back pain meant a very serious new complication; he asked for more demerol. Despite the fact that his therapist raised the dosage, Tom grew angry because he thought he was getting the "run-around" from the nurses regarding his medication. He complained that he was not receiving enough, and that the nurses were giving him aspirin instead of demerol. His tension and anger persisted, and he continued to complain of the pain. He lay in bed most of the time and began again to become depressed. His general behavior also changed. At times it was quite bizarre. He started to eat his meals standing up, complaining that the pain was so intense he was unable to sit down. Then he would sit down and complain that he was unable to stand up. He asked more and more for demerol, and his doctor increased the dosage. Still not satisfied, Tom presented new demands and schemes to his doctor in order to procure various analgesics and sedatives, in addition to the demerol that he claimed was not adequate to deal with his pain.

One month after the operation, Tom announced that the voices had started to bother him again while he was working at the occupational therapy shop. They said to him, "Get the hell out of here. You are bad." This disturbed him to such a degree that he refused to leave his room. Also, fearing to live alone, he stopped making plans for discharge from the hospital and his return to work. He said he knew that the voices were a sign of trouble, and he was unable to understand why his grip on things was slipping away from him. Soon after this he heard the voice of his old friend, and this depressed him very much because it made him realize how lonely he was; yet he made no effort to visit her. The more preoccupied with his auditory hallucinations he became, the more demanding were his requests for increased medication. At this time he was receiving 30 mg. of codeine sulfate every three hours, o.6 gm. of aspirin every three hours, and 120 mg. of sodium amytal at night. Four days later he was receiving 75 mg. of demerol instead of codeine every five hours. Then he was again changed to 45 mg. of codeine every three hours and was given in addition 1 gm. of chloral hydrate at night.

At this time Tom learned from one of the nurses that his psychiatrist was leaving the hospital because he was being inducted into the army. This was true, but the doctor had

preferred not to discuss his plans with the patient. Tom
reacted to it with a great deal of anger because he felt he
was being deserted again. He declared that he could not
face another loss, but he said nothing about this to his
therapist. Three weeks before his doctor actually left, he
told Tom about his prospective departure and drew a sharp
contrast between his own departure and that of Tom's first
psychiatrist. He also outlined a plan that he had worked out
with the visiting psychiatrist and the new resident who was
going to take over. Tom listened very quietly to all this,
and the only comment he made was that he thought the
overlap, as it had been called, between the time of his doctor's leaving and the new psychiatrist's arrival would be
very helpful. He then talked about the constant pain that
bothered him that day, just as if nothing extraordinary had
been discussed during the interview. When his therapist
suggested that he talk about the possible difficulties that
might arise from the change in therapists, Tom answered
that he wanted to get things over with as quickly as possible, but that he did not like to see things "broken up" in
so short a period of time. He also admitted that he had
already heard rumors that his doctor would be leaving the
hospital. He said that at first he did not want to think about
it and paid little attention, trying to forget, but then he
became annoyed and admitted that he had felt a great deal
of resentment and anger, which he was afraid to talk about.

After this interview, Tom was presented to the visiting
doctor. "If Dr. M. is not going to see me, he must be seeing
someone else who needs him more," Tom said. But as soon
as he had made this statement, he became upset and angry
and said he was being let down by his therapist. "I am torn
by such mixed feelings," he explained, but managed to end
the interview in a hopeful mood, saying he knew he was

going to get better and was planning to do everything he could to achieve this.

Interestingly, in another interview when he was again asked about his feelings concerning his doctor's departure, he denied completely that he cared in the least and compared it to the departure of his previous doctor, at which time he said he had felt absolutely nothing—"nothing bothered me at all." This denial alternated with a depressed mood, when he would say, "It is as if my arm is being cut off"; in his interviews he would remember having had nightmares about his "finger dragging on the ground." Once he said he was afraid he was going to have a delayed reaction. Following the departure of his first psychiatrist, it will be remembered, Tom developed an exacerbation of his ulcerative colitis that led to his readmission to the hospital.

Two weeks before the exchange of therapists, Tom went into a somewhat hypomanic stage, characterized by such statements as, "My spirits are up two hundred thousand percent." He spoke rapidly and became very active on the ward. He went to extremes, eulogizing his doctor and complimenting him on his "ability as a therapist," his "magnificent understanding of the patients," and his "tremendous self-restraint." In one interview he gave a long description of his fears of injury when he was younger, and he associated this with a fear of losing "a bone in his back" during his operation. He again expressed the conviction that something had gone wrong and that the surgeon had removed a piece of bone to repair the mistake he had made. He described this bone as being four inches long. When his therapist asked him to draw a picture of what he meant, he drew a picture of a penis; when asked to associate this, he said he remembered a voice describing "a lot of wafers piled on top of each other like a spinal column." He claimed that this voice had disturbed him during the first part of his admission to the psychiatry service while he was on the closed ward. He added that at times he was terrified because he knew that thoughts of this kind were meaningless and occurred only to insane people. He went on to describe what he thought the bones in the back were used for. Talking and gesticulating rapidly, he told how the bones opened and closed and how these movements had crippling and paralyzing effects all over the body. He continued to talk about how losing toys, missing bones, and losing his own doctor or something that was good for him were all connected in his mind and that he could not accept this possibility because it was the same as losing his uncle. At that point he broke into tears and began to describe his uncle's funeral. He said he had to bury his first doctor, but he could not tolerate the thought of burying the second one.

Following this interview, Tom became quite agitated and had to be transferred to the disturbed ward. He paced up and down. He talked somewhat incoherently about a friend named Bob, who had stood up on an iron beam, finally lost his balance, fell off, and injured himself very badly. As time went on, he grew more and more agitated and finally had to be sedated heavily for the night. The next day, although he appeared to be more quiet, he complained that he was all alone, that people did not want him, that they all moved away from him. Throughout the next week he continued to talk about being alone, but his hypomanic mood subsided considerably. He said, "When you are all alone and have to face someone new who will not understand you, then you get upset and tell him off." He added, significantly, "I am in hell because you're going away. I am sore at you because you have to go, but this is a terrible way to kick me around." His mood continued to change, and in a few days he started to become depressed. During this phase he paced the floors and was rude to the nurses and the other patients. He said that everything inside him wanted to let go, that he was tied up in knots, and that he felt there was something inside him trying to get out—because he was holding it back he was full of pain. His demands for medication increased again, and at times he became angry, threatening violence because his medication was withheld for ten or fifteen minutes after he had asked for it. He said he felt that people were letting him down right and left and that he really wanted to swear at or even to hurt others. That evening I met the patient for the first time.

CHAPTER IV

THE ENCOUNTER

TOM was a fairly tall, well-built man in his late thirties, with an intelligent face, blond curly hair, and blue eyes. The skin on his face was red and covered with pustules. He wore a hospital bathrobe and slippers. He shook my hand with a somewhat military gesture, straightening up his back and banging his heels together, but I noticed a sarcastic smile fleeting across his face. He said, "I understand you are an experienced doctor and know all about me. Well, Doctor, you have a great deal to learn." I said I agreed with him, because I was always interested in learning. He again smiled sarcastically. I added that I was starting work in July and expected to see him then.

He had an interview with his therapist after I left and immediately raised the question of medication, saying that his new doctor should be thoroughly indoctrinated in his needs. "There will be no monkey business. I must have my demerol. I insist on that." Later on, he talked about a fear of death that had come over him. He said he knew of two people who had had operations on the rectum. Their rectums had been removed surgically, like his own, and they were both dead in six months' time. Apparently he had heard a voice during the night that said, "You are going to die; the medication will carry you over for a while, but you must die." He went around seeking reassurance from the nurses and from other patients. He asked each person whether or not he knew of people who had had their rectums taken out and whether they were alive. Tom was becoming much more tense and talked to the nurses about wishing to murder the psychiatrist (his first) who had abandoned him and had moved away to open a "plush new office." But in the midst of all this he began to cry, saying that despite everything he loved his first doctor. He recalled that he had once told him he would like to commit suicide by eating pickles and peanuts and potato chips, which would make his ulcerative colitis worse, and that he wanted to die by eating something he liked very much. He said he had been neglecting himself, that he would not eat, and that this might be a good way to die—it would have been a way to punish his doctor who was worried about his diet and did not realize what his real problem was all about. The next day he gave a new reason why he had stopped eating. He said he felt that no one cared for him on the ward, that the nurses and patients antagonized him purposely, and that he was lonely for his little girl. Actually, when questioned further about this, he admitted that he had lost his appetite when his psychiatrist had gone away for a long weekend. He claimed that he had suspected something was going to happen to him and that his psychiatrist would leave him. He then added that, although he had lost his appetite, he wanted to eat in a "different way." When asked what he meant, he said he wanted to "eat medication." Actually, his sleeping medicine had been increased by the resident on duty on the previous night because the patient was unable to sleep and had complained about auditory hallucinations.

Tom's anger against the nurses for not giving him the "correct" medication increased, particularly when one of the night nurses asked him to prove to her that he needed it. When he tried to answer her, at that very moment he started to hear voices. He said that at first it was just a rumble rather than voices, but that actual voices soon followed and began to accuse him. He then described how he had gone around the ward gnashing his teeth and wanting to smash something. He had looked in at the occupational therapy shop and suddenly felt the urge to kill. He had hit and broken one of the table lamps because he wanted to smash "the dirty new doctor" who was assigned to him. The nurse became frightened and gave him what he asked for.

Tom became more agitated as the time for the exchange of doctors drew near. He again asked for a change in his medication, but his doctor refused. On the last day with his therapist, July 2, he staged quite a show. He dressed himself up and said he felt happy for the first time in a month. He did not mention the interview he had had with me the evening before. He talked about a dream: "There was a huge screen and I was trying frantically to get around it. I finally had to break it down because I couldn't move it, and there before me stood my uncle. I asked him for a drink and he opened up a bottle of whiskey with his mouth and gave me the bottle. I don't remember taking the bottle in my dreams, but I remember the profound satisfaction I felt." He associated having felt much stronger years ago after his uncle had given him the whiskey, and that this had meant the beginning of a new life at that time. He then told his doctor that in the last few days he had thought that everyone was trying to break him down, as he put it, by withholding medication for pain. He accused his doctor of being very cruel, particularly since this happened to be the last week he would be with him, but said he had forgiven him. Tom then expressed the wish to be hypnotized at this last interview, so that he could get rid of the "hidden things." He talked about how strong he was, how each of his arms had always been muscular and had helped him throughout his life. He said he could hit and kill with his left

fist anybody who dared him to. The night before, he went
on, his new doctor was introduced to all the patients around
the ward, but not to him. He said he hated his new doctor,
and he felt that nobody understood how dangerous he was
and that he was capable of destroying himself and others.
There was a great deal of anger in him that one day was
going to come out and overpower everybody, Tom continued, and he had to put up a terrific battle to keep it down.
Suddenly he stopped, looked at his doctor, and said, "The
interview is over. There is nothing more left." He got up,
shook hands, and departed. Later on, he was seen crying in
his room.

I took over the care of the patient, as well as of the ward,
on July 3. That evening I asked Tom to come to my office
for an interview. As soon as he entered the room, he started
to complain of pain in his coccygeal area and expressed anger
at the nurses because they had not notified me of the pain.
"The pain is terrible. I used to be strong and I could stand
it but I can't do it any more. I want to run away from pain.
It is like a bubble of air—sometimes it is here and then all of
a sudden it disappears." In more grandiose terms, he added,
"I used to be terrific in the way I could stand the pain. Once
I had an operation without anesthetic and I stood it. I
couldn't sit down for one whole year after that, but it made
no difference to me. Sometimes I felt sorry for myself, but
look at me now—I am afraid of the pain. There is anger
inside me and I want to kill. It all sounds crazy. Maybe I am
crazy. I had severe pain last night, but it's a little better now
that I'm here with you. There are so many things wrong
with me. I have infections and sores all over. I feel numb.
It all boils down to this pain problem."

DOCTOR: Could you describe the pain to me?
TOM: Well, I have a burning pain in my backside and a

throbbing pain as well. Then there's this itch all over. It also seems to burn at times. Do you want me to describe to you how it "radiates up and down" as you doctors call it? My Dr. M. thinks these pains are worse because of his impending departure. What do you think?

DOCTOR: I don't know. What about you?

TOM: I think he is wrong. He says this to cover up his guilt for leaving me, and I resent his interpretation.

DOCTOR: Guilt! Isn't it a strong word?

TOM: Of course not. He should feel guilty. No one can leave me without feeling guilty. Anyway, I never exaggerate, particularly when I'm complaining about the pain. You have a lot to learn about me, Doctor. I'm as bright as they come, and I've seen too many doctors. I know all their tricks and all their talk; I can tell a good one from a bad one right away. I know when the doctor is scared. I can read his face like an open book, and he better not lie about it. I can't stand lies. I can't stand my own lies neither, so I might as well admit it that Dr. M. is probably right and the pains are worse because he is going to leave me.

DOCTOR: I'm glad you admit it, if it is true, but I can see that you're upset and resent his departure. You also seem to be giving me a warning.

TOM: Wouldn't you? Dr. M. is a good doctor. He took good care of me. Anyone I get to know and like departs, and I am left all alone. It always happens to me. How would you feel?

DOCTOR: I understand how you feel, but we're not here to examine my reactions and my feelings.

TOM: So you are objective and scientific! I know! You don't care about me. You just do your job. I know your kind. I've seen many before. Well, Doctor, what's my diagnosis? [He glared at me angrily.]

DOCTOR: You exaggerate. I think we should concentrate

on you. I know and I want to stress the point that the good work which has been done between you and Dr. M. will not be wasted, and none of the benefits that have been gained will be lost. Dr. M. has talked to me at length about you and has told me he was confident about your future.

TOM: What is your diagnosis, Doctor?

DOCTOR: Come on now. You should know that I hope to be able to help you in my turn.

Tom smiled sarcastically, got up, and left my office, slamming the door after him.

The next day he greeted me with a barrage of angry curses, complaining of severe pain, and accusing me of not knowing anything about medicine or caring about him and of lying to him the day before. He said he knew that I had no intention of helping him out. "Do you understand what pain means?" he roared. I answered that I had some understanding of it, since I had experienced pain as something disagreeable, but I thought that reaction to pain or suffering varied from individual to individual. I added that, as far as I could see, he seemed to be suffering but that I was unable to assess just how much pain he had, and so the medication he was getting was on the basis of the amount ordered by his previous doctor. I said it might be difficult to eliminate the pain immediately, but I emphasized the fact that as a medical doctor I had a considerable knowledge of drugs. I said I felt confident that he, with my help, might be able to do something about the suffering and his reactions to it. He seemed to relax after this and talked about his worries and his recent fears that he was losing his grip. "In the last few days I've been lonesome. I've been thinking of my boys. Of course, I don't know what they think of me. Maybe they think I'm just a sick old guy. I also have the feeling that I work for a lost cause. I feel discouraged—it is a kind of desolate, flat feeling as if there was nothing, no hope. I don't like it. There is too much defeat. But I know there is a lot to be done if I only get rid of this pain. I would be satisfied with less money. I wouldn't ask for too much. I just want to live and be independent, but I always have this pain. I try to control it as much as I can but the more I think of it the worse it gets."

DOCTOR: I'm impressed by your efforts to overcome the pain. [Tom did not seem to pay attention to my remark.]
TOM: I've been fighting my battle for a long time. The other day—I wanted to hit someone that couldn't hit back. I always wanted to hit a woman. When I let go I want to burst the whole place open. I just want to kill and destroy. Yet when I'm with people I don't have any feelings like that. I'm angry only when I'm alone. I can never express such feelings. The voices had begun to return, particularly when I heard that Dr. M. was going to leave.
DOCTOR: Just try to describe the feelings.

He talked at great length about how he had been depressed at times and exhilarated on other occasions and how, following his operation, he had been very much worse psychologically because all his emotional symptoms had come back. I agreed that all this was probably connected with the departure of his therapist. As soon as I said this he flushed, and said he had known about it all along and that it was useless for me to repeat it; but he attempted to conceal his angry feelings from me, and almost succeeded. He again put on the sarcastic smile, which remained fixed on his face throughout the rest of the interview. It was apparent to me that he was depressed, tense, agitated, and preoccupied.

In his subsequent interviews with me he talked about marked hatred for the nurses, but said that what bothered him most was his inability to express such feelings. He also continued to complain about his pain, which he described to me in great detail, and talked about all the medication he needed to control it. "Once I was healthy too," he said with a smile, "but look at me now. This is the result of my aunt's doing." He flushed, clenched his fist, and added, "You can't imagine what powerful feelings I have in me."

TOM: I have been brought up to hate. What else could I do? No one ever cared about me. I had to stand for myself. Let me give an example. There was an old woman who lived around the corner from where we lived. One day she asked me to clean up her back yard which was full of all kinds of junk that had accumulated over the years. It was a heavy job, and it took me three days to do it, but I did a good job and the old lady was happy. She reminded me of my grandmother. She took me to her kitchen and gave me a glass of milk and some cookies. It was nice and warm in there. It was clean. My aunt's kitchen was always in a mess. After I ate all the cookies, the old lady gave me five dollars. I had never seen so much money in all my life. I kissed her hands and started to cry. She smiled and said, "Don't cry. I have other jobs for you and you can earn some more money." She gave me a whole jar full of cookies and several apples. When I went home my aunt was waiting for me. "Where have you been, you dirty brat?" she asked. This was always her greeting. "What have you got there? Whom did you steal the cookies and apples from?" I told her the story about the old lady, and like a fool I showed her the five-dollar bill. She quieted down right away. I could see she was pleased and you know what she did? She grabbed the money and the cookies and the apples from my hands and said, "Don't lie to me. I knew you stole them from her and the police will be after you. I'll keep the money for you." Of course, I never saw the money again, and do you know what she did with the cookies and the apples? She gave them to the kids that came knocking at the door that night, because it was Hallowe'en. I learned to hate her, and from then on I felt ready to kill people without the slightest remorse. When I start thinking in this way, however, I get frightened and I prefer to give up the fight and die rather than go on and on.

DOCTOR: Why suddenly do you become so discouraged when you feel so angry?

TOM: Because I can kill someone and then I'll end in jail.

DOCTOR: So it's the thought about the jail that stops you?

TOM: Not really. It's the thought that if I kill, I'll kill someone I need and I'll be left alone all over again. This is what frightens me most.

Two days later Tom came for his interview, holding a tangerine in his hand. He sat down quietly, looking me straight in the face without uttering a word. After several minutes of silence, he squeezed the tangerine fiercely and watched the juice run down over his clothes and onto the floor. Then, looking down, he said, "This tangerine is you because you want to bend me and destroy my will." When I attempted to find out what was bothering him, he explained that he had not received the type of medication he had expected. He related in great detail how angry he had felt about my interfering with the medication. This was his own province, he said. We had agreed that his previous therapist knew something about his condition, but I was useless and so he wanted to destroy me. I attempted to reassure him about the actual misunderstanding that had occurred and told him I thought his anger was displaced from the area that seemed to be foremost in his mind—the recent departure of Dr. M. and his anger at me and the nurses. I challenged him to talk openly about his feelings. I also agreed to discuss with him in advance any type of medication I was planning to give him or any change I contemplated. But I added that I was in charge of his medicines and that, though the medication was used to help him with his pain, it was helpless in altering his emotional reactions. The only way we could deal with his emotions would be by discussing them in psychotherapy.

At the time I took over the care of Tom, he was receiving the following medication for pain: 50 mg. of demerol every four hours, with two extra doses any time during the night; 0.6 gm. of aspirin every four hours; 1 gm. of chloral hydrate and 100 mg. of nembutal for sleep. Thinking all this exorbitant, I announced to him that a plan to cut down his medication from 50 to 40 mg. of demerol seemed to be a good idea. He was silent, but the next day he announced that he had had auditory hallucinations on the previous night that were a result of my plan to cut down the demerol. "It was Dr. M.'s voice that I heard whispering, 'Tom, I am leaving you.'" He said he had been reluctant to talk about the voices at first because he was afraid. He described them as not threatening but as clearer than they had been during the last week that his former doctor had seen him. I again tried to relate these hallucinations to the departure of Dr. M. He agreed that feelings of hostility and rage about Dr. M. had recurred and that he smashed the lamp next to his bed because on the face of the lamp was Dr. M.'s face and that he had lied to Dr. M. when he had said that smashing the lamp meant smashing me. He said he could not understand how such things could happen, and he realized that he actually wanted to destroy Dr. M. He remembered a dream: "Dr. M. was in front of a toy store. He watched the trains moving around and admired the other toys. Suddenly he got scared and started smashing things around. He destroyed everything. He even killed two people who worked in the store. He was caught finally and was put in jail. Soon, however, they let him go. You see he was insane. When I woke up the dream was in my mind. I thought that he was justified for killing everybody and destroying everything. I understand such feelings because I have similar ones. I know that when I reach my breaking point I can clear the whole place out in a minute—smash it all to bits. I want to get rid of this rage. I'm scared of my own anger. I think about it every minute of the day—all the time. It just goes around and around in my mind. When I'm angry I'm so unreasonable. My own thoughts are strong. I am the absolute master." He then looked at me for a long time and added, "You know, it was Dr. M.'s idea that you should be my psychiatrist. I didn't want you. I wanted Dr. R. who is so kind, but my doctor convinced me to have you because you are more experienced. Who cares if you know a lot? Can you cure my pain? Can you make me well? Can you give me back my rectum?"

During the next few days he described the voices as being of a whining nature, though he could hear very clearly at times his aunt's voice. He said, "I had a tough day yesterday, lousy. These whining voices make noises like a mosquito's hum, then they change into feminine voices. When they threaten me I get scared and worry, but they haven't so far. I can take it, don't you think so?" I said that I thought he could, particularly if he could cooperate in my plan to cut down his medication. He had seemed to be fairly comfortable up to this point, but suddenly he started to moan, saying that he was experiencing intense piercing pains. He actually became pale and perspired profusely. He begged me for more demerol. Although I suspected that this behavior was partly due to my cutting down his medication, I had no way of knowing how much pain he had; so I reluctantly agreed to increase his medication to 45 mg. of demerol. In the meanwhile, from the physical standpoint, the infection in Tom's rectal area seemed to be under control. Again, however, in the middle of an interview a few days later, he complained of excruciating pain and the inability to sit up. He said that the pain was the worst he had ever experienced and that he felt it was not associated this time with the departure of his previous therapist. I agreed with him and called the surgical service for consultation. Three large abscesses were lanced and drained, but the surgeons were skeptical about the value of such procedures, feeling that there were so many pockets of infection that, when one or two were opened, new abscesses were likely to appear later. They agreed that this was painful, so I decided to increase the patient's medication again from 45 to 50 mg. of demerol every four hours.

In the next few days Tom seemed to be somewhat improved, and on one occasion he entered my office, sat on my chair, and actually smiled. He was well dressed and well groomed. He said he had been thinking of Dr. M. because he knew he was a good doctor who had helped him a great deal. He added that he hoped I would do as good a job as Dr. M. had. I said it was up to both Tom and me to achieve that goal. He told me about a dream he had the night before, which was as follows: The head nurse was sitting with Tom in his room. He told her he knew that someone had to die, and she answered, "I know it too. It must be you." He repeated the dream to me three times, reading from a piece of paper on which he had recorded it because he was unable to recall the ending. Each time he read it he seemed to get more upset. He became very angry and finally said that he was now able to remember how the dream had ended. "I stacked a whole pile of newspapers very thick and tore them to pieces, ripping them all to small bits," he said. His asso-

ciations to the dream were that someone had to die of
separation from his doctor. He said that, just as he could rip
the newspapers, so he could rip women apart.

The next day he reported another dream to me. He had a
daughter who had died, and his grandmother was making
preparations for her burial. But when Tom looked at the
little girl he noticed that she was still alive. He asked his
grandmother what was happening, and she said, "Don't
worry, she's going to die very soon." But the baby opened
her mouth and laughed, and he noticed that her mouth was
full of orange juice. He became very tense and apprehensive
and refused to associate further to this dream. He switched
the subject and started to talk about his father's death when
he was two and a half years old. He remembered that his
brother, who was older than he, used to spank him because
he wet his pants. His mother always took his brother's side.
She also always gave cake and candy to his brother, but
never to him. He actually never got anything, he said. He
then went on talking about his uncle, who had a special
liking for his brother. He told me that he had always felt
like an outcast, and repeated the stories about his uncle and
aunt beating him unmercifully and how both of them
dressed him like a girl. He said he had told all this to his two
previous psychiatrists, but he felt I also should know. His
face relaxed when he talked about making peace with his
uncle but, despite this, the resentment at these experiences
continued in subsequent interviews.

During our next talk Tom suggested that his dream of
the day before demonstrated to him his murderous feelings
for all women, because he loved the little girl in the dream.
"If I have such murderous feelings for her, then I must be a
real murderer." He seemed to be shaken by this, but proceeded to discuss at length problems he had had with all
his children, describing how a social agency had recommended to him that he give them up for adoption.

"I remember it all very clearly. The elderly women came to my house and right away they started to explain to me that my children would be much happier if I consented to give my permission for their adoption. The younger of the two told me that they would make all the appropriate arrangements if I wanted them to do so. She talked and talked and I was getting more and more frightened. It looked all of a sudden as if it were my aunt talking to me. I could feel the same cold panic, the same shaking of my hands, the same knot in my stomach. My mind went blank and the next thing I knew I was hearing her ask me if I agreed. I nodded. She then started to tell me that I was wise because the children's happiness was of paramount importance. She went on and on. I could see her lips moving but I couldn't hear a word she was saying, and all I wanted her to do was to get out and never return. The only thing I could think of was that my aunt was standing there, talking to me. Suddenly she got out a piece of paper and put it on the table. She handed me her pen, 'Will you please sign down there on the dotted line?' I took the damned thing and I couldn't hold it. Then finally I started to sign my name very slowly. I just made the T and it was all wiggly, looking more like a J. I felt a cold sweat come all over me. Thoughts were racing through my mind. 'Why should I do what she wants me to do? I don't want to give my kids away, even though I know they will be better off. Why should I give them up?' All the time, however, a voice inside me kept on saying, 'You must do what she wants you to do, you must sign your name on the dotted line. You are no good and you know it, you were never any good. A spoiled brat! Do what the woman wants you to do. Sign your name.' I made the O of my first name. I knew all about that voice inside me. It was my aunt talking deep inside me, the way she had always talked, with hate, and with contempt. The lady was getting impatient. She said, 'Please go ahead and sign your name.

That's all you have to do.' I made a final effort. I scratched the M, but that was all. I turned and looked at her—my eyes must have betrayed my feelings. She moved back. I screamed at her at the top of my lungs, 'Get out! Get out of here, and leave my kids alone. I'll never give them up. Do you hear? Never!' She was frightened. Her friend got up and they both ran out of the room. Later on the priest came and told me that they had gone complaining to him. I got mad all over again, and I told him off. He was surprised but agreed that there was nothing to be done if I refused to listen to reason. It all boils down to something being taken away from me. I would lose something. It was the same as losing my rectum and my doctor and all the ones I loved. All my life I have been losing what I loved. Losing things is like pain—like a hurting inside. I feel I am torn apart. I feel there is a big hole inside me and it burns and burns and hurts inside."

His facial expression changed, and he started to cry. Later on that night he asked to see me. He told me he had felt very sad since the morning and wanted to ask me for some extra medication. He said that thoughts about his children were constantly in his mind.

The next day Tom again complained about the pain and asked for more medication. He refused to come to my office so I had to interview him in his room. He was moaning, "I can't take it any more. I can't be alone. It's too much for me. This thing is getting worse and worse." When I asked him to describe the pain he answered, "I feel like half way in hell. No one cares about me. I am alone on my deathbed." Then the following exchange took place:

TOM: It doesn't seem to make any difference.
DOCTOR: To whom?
TOM: I don't know.

DOCTOR: To me?

TOM: Sure. You don't care. How would you like it if I hit you under the belt?

DOCTOR: Do you want me to say "go ahead"?

TOM: Yes, but it wouldn't make any difference. You understand my trouble. It takes the fun out of it. Something always goes wrong. Everything is mixed up. Why does it always have to happen to me? I get all upset. Anyway, who cares? Life is meaningless and death is like a big dark room— a nice place to rest.

DOCTOR: But death doesn't solve any problems.

TOM: It solves all the problems. I don't deserve this pain. I know I don't. I think it's cruel to suffer so much. I hate to see myself in misery. I'd rather break my neck to prevent all this pain. Last night I felt sad and I wanted the nurse to get in touch with you. I had only a few minutes before my next medication was due. Each minute, however, was so terribly long. I asked for you. I almost went crazy. I wanted to bang my head against the wall. This is why I want to punch you. Here, I talk and talk but I don't say anything.

He seemed discouraged. His facial expression had changed, and he looked sad, pale, and crushed.

Again a few days later Tom claimed that the voices had returned and were more persistent than ever. He said he heard the voices of his boys calling him, begging him to take care of them, but he had not become too alarmed because the voices this time were not threatening. As the frequency of his auditory hallucinations increased, so did his demands for medication and his complaints about pain. He said he always felt frightened during the night because of thoughts that he feared might drive him to commit suicide. He begged to have more medication, and later on in the interview he angrily demanded more demerol.

At the departure of Mrs. N., one of the women patients

on the ward to whom he had become quite attached, Tom appeared to be extremely gloomy. He said that as soon as Mrs. N. left and the door was closed, he felt he wanted to smash, kill, and break things, and the thought of extra medication came immediately to his mind. He asked for more demerol, but promised he was not going to make any further requests for an increase.

In sum, the first month of my taking charge of Tom's care was a stormy one. Three main features emerged during our interviews: (1) The separation from his previous therapist appeared to predominate, and his ambivalence for him came out strikingly in his anger at me and his demands for increased medication; (2) although physically Tom was not in too bad a condition, the infections and the abscesses persisted, and the increase in the frequency and power of his auditory hallucinations was ominous; (3) his drug addiction was the major practical problem. I had tried to win the patient over, but felt more and more discouraged about the future.

CHAPTER V

THERAPEUTIC IMPASSE

AFTER a month in my psychiatric care, there was no evidence of improvement in Tom, and the problems we had faced all along persisted. His complaints of pain and demands for medication continued; his hostility toward me became much more pronounced; and in his general behavior on the ward he was getting even more difficult to manage. His physical condition also continued to deteriorate. The bloody foul-smelling discharge from several ulcerated areas around the anal region occurred more regularly, and the skin of the entire abdomen was inflamed. Cultures showed growth of various organisms: B coli, streptococci, and staphylococci were abundant. A series of abscesses had developed and, despite occasional drainage, became more numerous, as the surgeons had predicted.

The most alarming feature to me, however, was that I found myself losing interest in the case. A psychotherapeutic despair had set in. I felt that the treatment of this difficult and hostile patient, who had a complicated problem and who already had received many hours of psychotherapy without any evidence of help, could only end in failure. I felt that something extraordinary was required, but I was at a loss about the course to pursue. I considered the possibility of trying conventional treatments, such as insulin or electric shock, but I knew that this would not do because of his physical condition. I even considered psychoanalysis, although I realized that such treatment would be impracticable. I continued to see the patient daily, but after each interview I was more convinced of my inability to help Tom understand the nature of his emotional conflicts.

In the meanwhile, Tom continued to talk about his separation from his previous psychiatrist and from Mrs. N., the discharged patient whom he considered his friend. He saw everything in terms of separation. For example, he said that when the barber's razor came close to his neck when he was having his hair cut, a numbness would develop, followed by an uncontrollable trembling from the fear that his head would be "chopped off," just as he had been chopped off from his former therapist. When he talked about getting used to the ileostomy, he described a dream in which he felt that the ileostomy bag caused him to be different from other people, but as soon as he was separated from the bag he would become panicky; when he put it back on, he felt normal again.

TOM: Most of the time, however, I have a terrific resentment at the ileostomy bag. In the last two nights I had dreams, but the bag was missing and I was intact. Lately I can't accept this damned thing.

DOCTOR: But it serves an important purpose, as you know.

TOM: Of course I know. I used to be so sick that I was glad to have the operation. Before whenever I'd discover blood in my stools I'd think that my life was pouring out of me. A few days postoperative the surgeon came to my room and tried to put a bag on me. I was bewildered. All of a sudden a bag. No explanation—no nothing. I thought, my guts are gone so the pain is gone, but with this bag on I feel ashamed.

DOCTOR: Is there anything you can do to improve it?

TOM: That's the first intelligent thing you've said. Sure I have ideas—plenty of ideas. I'll make "the perfect ileostomy bag."

The next day he brought to the interview a drawing of an ileostomy bag.

TOM: It's a good one, don't you think?

DOCTOR: It looks efficient.

TOM: What do you know of bags?

DOCTOR: I know very little about them.

TOM: Well, it's not a joke. I'm interested in attending ileostomy-bag class.

DOCTOR: Do you want me to make arrangements for you to go?

TOM: I can do it myself. I had a dream last night. I was walking all alone on the beach when suddenly a pirate came at me with a huge sword. He started to cut me up. I could see pieces of my flesh all over the sand but I felt no pain. I started to laugh. He stopped and looked at me bewildered. He said, "Doesn't it hurt?" But I kept on laughing. I grabbed him by the throat, but suddenly he turned into a woman. I felt paralyzed. I let him go and he ran away.

DOCTOR: What associations do you have to this dream?

TOM: The pirate reminded me of the priest who tried to get me to go back to my family after I ran away. You know all about that, don't you?

DOCTOR: Yes, I do. What about the priest?

TOM: Well, he threatened me. He said I would be in serious trouble and I argued with him. I proved to him that there was nothing he could do to scare me. I held my own, yet he was a college-educated man. Deep inside I was so mad at him I could have killed him. He never knew the misery I had been through, the deep resentment, the attacks of rage and hate that I feel at myself.

DOCTOR: Why did the pirate turn into a woman?

TOM: It's my aunt. I don't know what to do with women.

DOCTOR: So your anger is really at women?

TOM: Maybe you've got something there.

DOCTOR: If one is angry at the right person, one doesn't have to be so angry at oneself.

TOM: What's my diagnosis, doctor?

DOCTOR: You changed the subject. Why do you ask?

TOM: Well, am I crazy, doctor?

DOCTOR: I know that you have ulcerative colitis. I know that you have pain and that you suffer a great deal. I know that at times you're very angry. These are my observations. Furthermore, I don't think you like me.

TOM: You bet your life I don't.

In his interviews he continued to express a great deal of anger at having to wear the ileostomy bag; yet he gave much thought to how he might improve its construction. He had some good ideas, and I continued to encourage him to work on them in the occupational therapy shop, where materials would be given him to experiment with. In later interviews he discussed at length the improvements he had invented for the bag, but he finally became disappointed with his ideas because he felt he would never be able to make "a perfect bag because he was not perfect himself."

His resentment at the other patients on the ward, as well as at the nurses, continued to soar. He recounted a dream in which he was sitting at a round table, with a head nurse on his right and several other nurses on his left. He seemed to be the judge and announced that someone had to die. He wrote the death sentence on a piece of paper and passed it around. Then he got up and announced that he was going to kill someone. He held a newspaper in his hand and ripped it to pieces, adding, "This is what I am going to do to your nurses."

In another interview he talked about his old friend, who had not written to him, and he said he felt deserted by her.

He also felt deserted by Mrs. N., who had not returned to visit him. In one interview he was particularly disturbed. "Voices" had bothered him so much the previous night that he had been unable to sleep. He said one of the voices was that of another woman patient whom he liked very much. He said he had recently tried to establish a relationship with this woman, but that she seemed uninterested in him. He realized, he added, that whenever he came close to people, threateningly angry feelings would immediately be aroused in him and those feelings would drive people away. At another time he said it was difficult for him to discuss this woman patient with me, but he refused to give me his reasons for this. When I encouraged him to talk freely, he said that recently he had felt an interest in her, but he could not explain why. "I don't want to talk about it any more. It's simply a conviction that I can help this patient. That's all." He also said he felt uncomfortable about being the only man on the ward.

The next day he received a postcard from another woman patient who had been discharged from the ward, and he was very happy about this, though he wished the card had been from Mrs. N. But the more he talked in positive terms about the women patients, the angrier he became at his mother, who still had not come to visit him. He said this should not be bothering him because he had ceased to care for her, and, besides, whenever he came close to a woman, he inevitably got hurt. The next time he saw me, he asked for a leave of absence for the weekend; but he soon realized how completely dependent he was on his medication, withdrew his request, and started to cry.

In the next interview he looked haggard and said he felt depressed, let-down, and guilty. He could not understand why anybody would put up with him: "I am no man, with this ileostomy bag. I should be shot." When I tried to find out the reason for this extreme condition, he answered that it was because he was "all rotten inside." He said that he had felt almost ready to go home but then quickly realized that he could not, and the anger and depression had returned.

In another interview he described a dream about his father, who was sitting quietly and failed to recognize Tom when he approached him. Tom then realized that the man in his dream was not his father at all but his own self, with a mustache. When he awoke, he was terrified with thoughts about death, and he felt that he had dreamed himself dead.

Throughout this time, Tom's complaints of pain continued to increase. He was seen again by the surgeons, and because he insisted on knowing the exact nature of his condition he was told that he had a chronic infection of his anal area. As soon as the surgeons left, he asked for medication because, he said, he had developed murderous feelings for the surgeons as well as for the people in his past. He said he was afraid he might kill someone, and he described two instances when he had felt a great urge to kill his boss, whom he thoroughly disliked. On both occasions, it happened that his boss had been unkind to him, had criticized his work, had told him he looked thin, and had said, "If you can't do this work you must be sick."

He continued to complain of constant pain which made him unable to concentrate, unable to go to occupational therapy, and unable even to talk. It turned his life into a nightmare, he said. He also continued to complain about the voices. "When I was in bed yesterday, I heard echoes. It was a little boy talking to me. Then I thought I recognized the voice of one of my boys. I tried to ignore it. The voices became louder and told me that I should write to my children. I tried to read but I couldn't. I worry because I'm afraid that my mind is playing tricks on me. Before I used to like to hear voices but now I'm frightened. Last night I heard a plane go over the hospital and then I heard the voices clearly. I thought maybe it had something to do with my interview with you. I kept on trying to think of something else, but it didn't work. Then I started thinking of suicide—and I mean real suicide, no foolish stuff, real suicide! The future is black. I have no one—nothing. I keep on thinking I'm no good. I think I'll find peace in death." "It may be so," I said, "but I think you're trying to impress me."

TOM: You're damned right I'm trying to impress you. For a week now I've been trying to tell you that I'm lonely, but you don't understand. No one does.

DOCTOR: Do you think I'll understand if you commit suicide?

TOM: You'll be sorry then, and all the others too.

DOCTER: Maybe some people will, but that's not a way to go about making friends. Suicide is the loneliest act in the world.

TOM: You may be right, but when I feel the way I do I want to hurt others, including you. At least they will feel some pain, the same way I do.

He suddenly began to accuse me of deliberately cutting his interviews short while he had been trying to put his whole self into the talks. For that reason he hated me: he thought I was taking away something that belonged to him, and this always created a great deal of pain for him. He continued to make many demands for medication and tested me in every conceivable way, because, as he had said, he was unsure of me and despised me. "I have hated you ever since the first time I saw you. You are the worst doctor I have ever met," he told me. My attempts to calm him down were of no avail. Nothing seemed to satisfy him.

On the morning following this interview, I was told by

the assistant resident on duty that Tom had been extremely angry the night before and was threatening to kill me. When I went to him for his interview he was in a frenzy. He paced the floor; he told me he had taken a pot of flowers that was near his window and had broken it to pieces the previous day. He said he had forgotten why he was so angry, and when I mentioned that he had felt I had cut our interviews short, he denied it, saying that he really did not remember. Then he stared at me and said, "You implied that I needed another operation so as to keep me here in the hospital indefinitely until I become completely dependent on you." It is true that I had mentioned the possibility of further surgery, but I had never suggested that he should stay in the hospital indefinitely, which seemed to be what he wanted. I also acknowledged that I had had my difficulties with him and that I might have welcomed his temporary transfer to the surgical service. He said he definitely did not want another operation and then appeared to calm down. "At least you're honest," he said.

The deterioration in Tom's physical condition persisted. Large carbuncles began to develop on his face. His chest wall now became inflamed, and his rectal discharge increased despite several sitz baths a day. He also continued to complain about the auditory hallucinations and the severe pain, and his demands for medication became even more frequent. On several occasions I felt that Tom could no longer be trusted on the open ward; at the same time, I feared that he might interpret any move to have him confined in the closed ward as hostility on my part, and he might become even more uncooperative. So I decided to leave him where he was, but to have him watched constantly because of his impulsive behavior. As his hostility toward me increased, he expressed discouragement about his progress. I, in turn, felt utterly discouraged about the whole situation and became convinced that Tom should be transferred either to the surgical service or to a mental state hospital.

At this point I became completely aware of a punitive attitude on my part, and I discussed the matter with my supervisor. We agreed that Tom was not responding to psychotherapy; in addition, both the medical and surgical services found that his physical condition was becoming progressively worse in spite of the fact that everything possible was being done for him. His infections continued to spread, and the antibiotics seemed to do no good. Some of the organisms responsible for the infections were resistant to these antibiotics, and thus, whenever the patient was treated with one, a new infection would flare up from an organism that was resistant to the drug being used. We decided, then and there, that something drastic must be done.

It seemed clear to us that the patient's fundamental difficulty was his inability to trust anyone emotionally. Having seen the people with whom he had been most involved die or desert him—his father, his grandmother, his uncle, his two psychiatrists—he was afraid that he might hurt, or perhaps kill, any person to whom he found himself attached emotionally. He also feared that he himself might be hurt or harmed by such a person. Loss and separation were frightful experiences that had happened repeatedly during his life. The only hope left to us was to attempt to convince him that, for the first time, he could depend on and completely trust a human being, that it was possible for him to have a relationship with someone without fearing that dread loss. But how could one achieve such a result? After all, we had been doing our best to help Tom for a long period of time. Something not only drastic but dramatic had to be tried. As a last resort, we thought of establishing an anaclitic (from the Greek "to lean on") relationship. After thorough consideration, it seemed most appropriate to this patient's need.

Anaclitic treatment involved a plan to satisfy all of Tom's desires and needs, possibly for the first time in his life, in a final attempt to convince him that he could trust his therapist. So it was decided that the patient should be encouraged to regress to the point of complete dependence on me, and that I should be the one to see that his wishes were fulfilled. After a period of entire dependence on his part, and reassurance and support from me, we hoped he would be convinced emotionally of my good will; following this we planned slowly to restrict his privileges and to encourage him to become more self-reliant.

I realized that such a treatment necessitated a complete change in my attitude. An enormous amount of effort would be required to satisfy this extremely demanding and hostile patient. In addition, such an approach would require a major change in policy by all concerned: the nurses, the dietitians, the other residents, and even the other patients. Not only did we need the permission of the chief of service to undertake such a radical program, but we needed the cooperation of other services. Anaclitic treatment involved not only satisfying the patient's every request in terms of food and other such items, but also in terms of medication. And, above all, it would require emotional support of this patient on my part, on a twenty-four-hour basis. This was the challenge I had to face. I was frankly apprehensive about it, although my supervisor assured me of his support and the chief of service gave his permission to proceed. Even with all of this encouragement, I still doubted my ability to work in such a manner and to give so much of myself to a patient who hated me. But there was no other alternative, and I decided to go ahead with the plan.

The next day I went to see Tom and announced to him,

somewhat dramatically, that we had decided to start on an entirely new kind of treatment, which, to my knowledge, had not been tried before. I then asked him to come over to the head nurse's office with me. I told him, in her presence, that from then on he could have whatever he wanted and that all he had to do was simply ask for it. The head nurse was as unconvinced about the ultimate success of this treatment as I was, but she tried to be cooperative. Tom looked perplexed and utterly incredulous. He said he felt doubtful about the plan and admitted that he could not believe it would work. "There must be a catch to it," he said. After all, he knew that both the head nurse and I hated him. What if he asked to have a steak, for example, or the lobster meat that he liked so much? Would we give it to him? I told him to ask and find out. Still disbelieving, he said, "Could I have a steak for lunch, Miss M.?"

"How do you like it, Tom, rare or well done?" she answered. This was the beginning of the anaclitic treatment.

CHAPTER VI

THE ANACLITIC
RELATIONSHIP

BEFORE I go into the anaclitic relationship as such, it might be useful to describe my attitude toward the patient during all this time. Originally I had accepted with hesitancy the notion of anaclitic treatment for a patient who was extremely disturbed, unpredictable, and hostile. In addition, his physical condition was precarious. Since I had no experience with such a treatment, I thought that a more orthodox approach—a more conservative one—might have a better chance of success. During my first two months with Tom, psychotherapy did not seem to help. He complained more and more about his pain and demanded more and more medication; he also was depressed, agitated, and angry; and he made it clear to me at every opportunity that I was unable to help him.

When we decided that anaclitic treatment was to be tried, I realized that the additional demands placed on me would require a complete change of mind. I questioned my ability to give him all he wanted, and I doubted very much the possibility of obtaining a successful result. In addition, I realized that, when I thought of the nurses' being hostile to the patient, I was looking around for ways to avoid giving this anaclitic therapy. It was certainly true that Tom had worn thin their patience with his incessant sarcastic and derogatory criticism. I also remembered what the head nurse had told me about the unwillingness of the nurses to go along with such foolishness, and that only if they were ordered to would they cooperate. As a result of these thoughts, I had two talks with the head nurse, the dietitian, and the occupational therapist, and explained to them the plan of treatment and the rationale behind it. I did admit to them that I had serious doubts about this technique, but I heard myself saying that it was a new and fascinating approach, which to my knowledge had not been tried before, and I even appealed to their sense of adventure. Following these interviews, I was convinced that my own crisis was past. It turned out to be premature wish fulfillment on my part. But this was the turning point, and I decided to proceed with the anaclitic treatment.

In a second meeting, the nurses agreed to give me their assistance. That was all I had hoped for originally, and I was satisfied. I promised to have frequent meetings with them in the future, to review together our ideas about the patient's progress. Very satisfactory conferences were held throughout the period of the patient's regression; but when he started to become unmanageable, the old fears and apprehensions in the minds of the nurses were again awakened —but more about this later.

Throughout this period I was lucky to have the strong support and encouragement of my supervisor, whom I saw on a weekly basis. These sessions helped me greatly. What disturbed me most, however, was the possibility that the patient would make such overwhelming emotional demands on me that I would not have any time left to deal with my other duties and my primary responsibility—the running of an active psychiatry ward in a general hospital. Despite all my misgivings, I began to be fascinated by this new approach, and the patient seemed to be more trustful of me and willing to cooperate. Realizing that every possible effort had to be made to help Tom learn to deal with people emotionally in a new way, I knew that this was the time to support the patient to the utmost. He could not be abandoned, and the realization of the magnitude of my responsibility affected me deeply. I knew that Tom's depression was a reaction to the loss of vital, key people in his life—the very few people he had been able to feel close to, those who liked him and whom he needed to depend upon because of his own incapabilities, weaknesses, and helplessness. Suddenly I began to feel happy at the opportunity to try anaclitic therapy.

My change in attitude was reflected by my going to visit Tom immediately. I found him in fairly good spirits. He said he would do all he could to help me. In subsequent interviews the content of his communications did not change very much, but what was strikingly different was his attitude toward me. From a hated person whom he viewed as having taken over the place of his "beloved therapist" and one who was trying to deprive him of his medication, I became, practically overnight, someone who he felt was trying to be on his side—someone who had offered a different way to approach his problems. Tom knew only too well that the approach had not been tried before, and he seemed to feel important because of it; temporarily his self-esteem was elevated.

He now talked a great deal about his dreams. "There was some food, and I did not know how to get rid of it. I threw two apples into a sewer and felt a very severe pain." He associated to this dream the departure of the two therapists who had "abandoned" him. He felt frustrated because he could not give anything to anyone for fear that the recipient would take it away and leave him alone. The only thing he could give was "pain." "I am unable to have a bowel movement because of the ileostomy and I feel angry because it keeps reminding me that I am half-human." Although he was upset by this dream, he still felt there might be some hope. He went on:

TOM: Why does this pain last so long? It stays on and on and it gets me all confused, all excited, and then I get to do foolish things.

DOCTOR: So your reaction to the pain is the biggest problem?

TOM: In a way, yes. There's a lot to be done about this reaction. I try to control my reactions as much as I can, but at times the more I think of it the worse it gets.

DOCTOR: I know you're fighting a difficult battle.

TOM: [with a smile] Yes, I've been making a lot of effort for a long time, and I know I still have a spark left in me. You try to figure this one out. I had a funny thought the other day. I always wanted to hit at something that couldn't hit back at me, like a punching bag. My aunt came to my mind. When she was alive I wanted to let go. I just wanted to kill her, to destroy her, to wipe her off the face of this earth, but the funny thing is that when I was with her I had no feelings at all.

DOCTOR: You deny your feelings when you're with women.

TOM: You doctors always say this, but what can I do? If only I could get rid of this rage. I'm scared of my own fury. It just comes out of nowhere. I used to be so mad at you I could kill you, but I feel so much better about you lately. You're a good doctor. I want you to know that when I get mad everything must be mine. I want to bend your will to mine. My thoughts are absolute—but such power doesn't give me any satisfaction. My life has always been full of rage, no love, no fun, just pain.

DOCTOR: I do understand you.

TOM: Lately, on the other hand, I feel deep inside me that

I might be able to control this rage. It has a lot to do with my liking you all of a sudden. Where does all this good feeling come from? You seem to have changed overnight. From the devil you became the angel.

DOCTOR: I haven't changed much, but you seem to have changed a great deal since we started this new treatment.

TOM: I guess so, but it's hard to say.

DOCTOR: Do you think this new attitude is going to last?

TOM: I think it will.

Tom's behavior in relation to the other patients on the ward also seemed to improve. He became outwardly friendly with several of them and announced that he was giving them psychotherapy. When I pointed out that he was identifying with me in this respect, he smiled. "But you can't treat them all, Doctor. You must treat only me," he said. He told me also that he was able to help three patients on the ward by giving them support and reassurance. He said he was a better psychiatrist than the surgeons because he supported other patients; the only thing the surgeons talked to him about was the ileostomy bag, and he took this to mean that there was not much hope for him.

He continued along in this way for several days, maintaining himself on the same medication he had been taking before. He talked about the medication frequently.

TOM: One of your surgeons came to see me last night.

DOCTOR: My surgeons?

TOM: Yes, the smart ones who are always in a hurry and spend just a couple of minutes with me.

DOCTOR: What's this all about?

TOM: Well, I showed him an abscess I have on my back. He poked around and around and then he said that he'd be back to look at it again. "Don't worry," he said, "I'll keep an eye on you." You see, I know what that means.

It means that he'll be back in two or three weeks—maybe a month.

DOCTOR: Come on now, you know this isn't true.

TOM: Well, anyway I was mad. My fist doubled up when he said it. I hit the pillow softly. Later on I felt ugly and I asked for some medication. I realize I asked for it because it soothes my anger, but what can you do? I truthfully did not have any pain when I asked for it, but it did the trick for me. I felt better.

DOCTOR: Tell me how it happened.

TOM: I'll tell you, at first, right after the shot, when it had no time to act I started thinking of nice things.

DOCTOR: Such as what?

TOM: Well, vacations, beautiful places by the seashore. I remembered my grandmother telling me a story about the old country when she was a little girl. It was a nice spot by the water, with beautiful dark green pine trees all around. It was warm, summertime I guess. The sea was calm, nothing stirred. She used to lie down on the beach and look at the mountains far away. When it got dark she would gaze at a sky full of stars. One night a man came and sat next to her. He wanted to make love to her but she was too fine, too good, too beautiful. He didn't dare to touch her. It's a sad story in a way.

DOCTOR: The ending of the story is yours, isn't it?

TOM: How did you know?

DOCTOR: I think you were that man, Tom. I know you loved your grandmother.

TOM: That's so long ago. You're right, Doc. It had a different ending—something to do with being late and getting a spanking. I don't remember.

DOCTOR: It makes no difference. Now what about the medication?

TOM: Well, this story made me think of other good

things. I soon started feeling tired. I knew the medication was working. I fell asleep.

DOCTOR: So it was your fantasy that soothed your anger, wasn't it?

TOM: I guess so. Yes, it did. You see, it's like this. There are two sides to me. There is an intelligent, good, rational understanding side, and there is a cruel, unreasonable, nasty part to my nature.

DOCTOR: All of us are like that. What counts is to recognize and learn to live in peace with both sides.

TOM: It's worth fighting to achieve that and we can do it together. [He was silent for a while and then, smiling, he went on.] I had another funny dream and debated with myself whether I should mention it to you or not. I decided finally you should know. I was in your office. Two huge desks were next to the door. I sat behind one and you sat behind the other. My desk was fancier than yours. One by one the ward patients came in. Even Mrs. N. was there. I asked my friend, "Who is your doctor?" and she said that I was. I asked all of them the same question, "Who is your doctor?" and each one answered, "Tom, you are my doctor." Then I told them to come and sit next to me. All the women chose me as their doctor. I felt sorry for you, Doc, so I asked the head nurse to come in. I asked her, "Who is your doctor?" and she said that you were the one. So I said, "Fine, you go and sit next to him." She came close to you, but you got up and said, "Oh no! Tom is my doctor," and you came and sat next to me. All the patients roared. That was the end of my dream.

DOCTOR: Well, what do you think about it?

TOM: It's obvious! I beat you in your own game.

DOCTOR: Why did you hesitate to talk to me about it?

TOM: You see, sometimes I think I can be a hell of a good psychiatrist, even better than you and you're one of the best. It may take years of medical training that I don't have, but it takes something else. One must be very sensitive to suffering himself in order to be able to understand others.

DOCTOR: This may be so, up to a certain extent.

TOM: Well, anyway, I hope you don't mind this competition.

DOCTOR: Not in the least.

Tom smiled and left the room. When I encountered him later in the corridor, he started to laugh and said, "Don't take me too seriously, Doc; I like to make jokes sometimes."

DOCTOR: So you think my feelings were hurt?

TOM: Yes. After all, in my dreams all the girls chose me. You can't beat that, can you?

DOCTOR: I guess I can't.

"O.K., you're a good loser," he said, and went to the occupational therapy room where five female patients were busily at work.

In other interviews he talked about his sexual feelings for some of the woman patients on the ward and expressed a certain amount of anxiety about his being the only male patient. But such feelings did not last long. He would soon change the subject and talk with pride about his conquest of women. He mentioned a female ward patient who seemed to be interested in him. "Last night her husband came to visit her. He kept on looking at me in a queer way, and later on the same thing happened. I thought, I bet he's thinking that I'm having an affair with his wife. Before he left he came over to me and said that he thought we had gone to school together. I was disappointed." After this, Tom related that when he was a little boy the children did not want to have anything to do with him. When he was in grade school, he was shy with girls but seemed to become more popular when he grew up.

In another interview he talked with much feeling about another female patient who was discharged. He had liked to talk to her and to hear all about her problems. He went on: "Before she left she told me that I had helped her more than her own doctor. She gave me a kiss. It meant so much to me. It made me feel big and strong. Little things like that make a world of difference."

In the next interview he talked about a male patient who had just been admitted.

TOM: He starts to play the piano and my whole mood changes—too much noise! I get two pillows and a magazine and go into the bathroom to take a bath. I rested well, but I was irritated when I saw him again. I want no competition. I want all the women to myself.

DOCTOR: You're exaggerating.

TOM: Well, when I was young, as you know, I had a tough time but I was able to use my brains, and I managed to do pretty well. I earned a lot of money, but, you know something, I could never understand women. Lately I feel somehow different, more confident about women— even the nurses don't bother me so much. All seems to be going along fine. Yet I have the feeling that you disapprove.

DOCTOR: I disapprove! Why?

TOM: Well, it's funny. I think you're jealous when the girls like me. Maybe this sounds silly, but I have the same notion about this other fellow, the new male patient.

He changed the subject and mentioned that lately he had been comparing me with Dr. M. "No one was able to bring out of me so many different things as you were able to do, Doctor. We have a good glimpse of what goes on and it makes me happy. I used to be terribly afraid of my angry feelings, particularly when I thought of killing people. I remember a friend of mine I wanted to shove in front of a train. I could see him being hit by the engine. I had a tremendous urge to push him, but I didn't do it. I don't know why I think of such unpleasant thoughts when I tell you that I have a good feeling about you." He again mentioned his operations. "They created havoc with me. I went through hell, and I never got rid of the pain. I have trouble after trouble." He again described in detail his relations with the surgeons. When I pointed out to him that he was avoiding something by changing the subject, he admitted that he was doing it on purpose because he did not want to give me the idea that he liked me and was becoming dependent on me. I invited him to talk more about this, but he refused.

The next day Tom seemed more upset. He related a terrifying dream. "I was in a bathroom trying to have a bowel movement; blood was pouring out of me. I said to myself, 'Tom, there goes your life. You should flush your life away, down the toilet bowl.' " He associated to his postoperative days when the surgeon came to show him how to wear an ileostomy bag. He remembered being bewildered and angry at the surgeon for offering no explanation. "It was like the blood pouring out of me in the dream, but then I started thinking. I said to myself, 'Your guts are gone so the pain will be gone.' I felt happy, but this thought didn't help much because when you wear a bag you're abnormal. You're no good." The next day he related another dream about the female patient who had given him a kiss. She had returned to visit him: "She came and sat on my bed and said that she was going to marry me. I was elated! My spirits are like a ladder, going up and down all the time. I feel fine this morning." With great pride he described how unpopular the other male patient was with all the women on the ward. "He is drawing pictures and shows them to the girls. He said the girls think he's sexy. He is not. He looks like hell, even though he managed to talk to Miss C. You know, Doc, she told me that she was scared of him. I have my eyes open. When he makes remarks about the girls I want to throw an ashtray at him. I told him to stop making a fool of himself. I told him that Miss C. is a sick girl, and with his talk he could make her crazy. I said I was going to complain to you about it because you were the chief. You see, the girls bring their troubles to me. They should bring their troubles to their doctors, but I guess they like me and I help them. I say to them, 'If you talk to your doctors the way you talk to me, everything will be all right.' You know, at first no one liked you. I sure hated your guts because you were the chief, but now everybody seems to be on your side.

DOCTOR: Now you're paying me compliments.

TOM: Sure I pay you compliments. You're the best God-damn doctor in the world. I like you because you always hit the nail on the head. Look what you're doing to me. I feel physically better and I've gained a great deal of weight during the last week.

DOCTOR: I'm very pleased with your progress.

TOM: My spirits are one hundred percent better. I'll give you an example. I feel more self-confident. Even my night-mares don't frighten me. I had one last night. It was all about the war. I was in a tank racing against the enemy. Our side was winning, when all of a sudden as my tank was entering into a small village an old woman started to swear and scream at me. "There is no return," she said, "All of you will die." I woke up in a cold sweat, but I figured it out. I had the dream because of a book I'm reading about the war. *Signed with Honor* is the title. Excuse me just a minute.

He got up and left my office. He soon returned with a book in his hands, which he placed on my desk.

DOCTOR: I didn't know that you like to read books.

TOM: Oh yes, I read during the night. Sometimes I stay up all night. I noticed that you like books too. You have quite a collection in here. They're not all medical books either.

DOCTOR: There's nothing better than good books with new ideas. They can take you to new places and open up wide horizons for you.

TOM: I saw this book *The Possessed* open on your desk. Is it a good one?

DOCTOR: It's one of the best books I have ever read. I'm rereading it now.

TOM: What's it about?

DOCTOR: About evil. It describes life in Russia during the last century. It also deals with politics and revolutions. There are some very interesting characters. There is a very independent and good man, several foolish fellows who do what they are told, a cold, proud, sick aristocrat, and a scheming, selfish, malignant friend of his. Finally, there is a man who believes he has the right to kill himself, and does, while others take advantage of his act to murder the good man.

TOM: What a story! That's my kind of stuff. I'd like to read it.

DOCTOR: You may borrow it any time you want.

TOM: Another thing I wanted you to know about: I'm

making a cartoon scrapbook. It will be good for a sick patient. This will be my kind of psychiatry. I'm sure it will help someone.

DOCTOR: I'd like to see it.

Tom departed in good spirits, and for the next week he seemed to be quite happy and contented.

CHAPTER VII

REGRESSION

THE INITIAL good period did not last very long. One day, a month and a half after we had started the treatment, Tom came to my office and announced that he had awakened at five in the morning because of a severe burning pain in his back. He had not asked for any medication because he knew what the pains were all about: "They are associated with losing someone you love, and you do not want to accept it." This thought had occurred to him while in bed and was followed by acute pain; but he decided to "chew it over with the doctor tomorrow," and he found out to his surprise that this thought seemed to help for a while and that the pain was much better. But later in the same interview, he started to cry because he remembered a woman patient who was discharged from the ward the day before. "Thoughts like these always made me feel like a child wishing for someone to put his arms around me and give me some consolation; but I can cry myself dry and no one cares, nobody comes to see me, this is how it always happens. I am always left alone." Despite these feelings, Tom managed to conduct himself well for two more weeks.

With me he tried to be friendly—even when he had to complain. "The nurses delay giving me my shots, Doc. You give me all you have and they take it away from me. My whole rectum has been removed and there is nothing left but a smelly bag. The nurses are tearing things away from me. Only women can do such things. My aunt did it and I was completely helpless—completely unable to fight her. I just sat there taking it." While this passive attitude became more and more pronounced, I noticed that his dependence on me was increasingly strong. In one talk during this two-week period, he complimented me on my "complete understanding" of his problem, "better than anyone else" had understood him in the past, and he contrasted me with the nurses who took things away from him and whom he wanted to smash. At this point he started to cry and make a peculiar whining noise with his tongue.

In a little while he began to talk again, saying he did not believe that his rectum was gone because at times he had a vivid notion that he was still complete. He associated this with weird fantasies of a "long tube divided into two parts, one side bleeding and painful, and the other always healthy and strong." He added, "The pain reminds me that my rectum is still there, and the medications take it away because the pain goes away. I know I'm taking too much medication. I want to cut it down, but I also feel that I'm glad my rectum was cut off." He then recounted how he decided to have his operation because he felt so miserable, was in constant pain, with his rectum discharging more and more pus day after day until finally his doctor told him that unless he got rid of his rectum he would die. "I figured I'd better die than go mad, but I soon changed my mind because I couldn't stand the pain." He remembered that when he awoke after the ileostomy he felt fine, but the thought immediately occurred to him that now he would go mad. He remembered being drowsy from the narcotic, yet still having a terrific backache. Weird ideas were always in his mind about bones being cut off and nerves being removed. When he woke up completely, he was sure he had been crippled and that he would have something wrong with him for the rest of his life.

Suddenly Tom stopped talking, walked up to me, pulled his shirt open, showed me his chest, and said, "Look, Doctor, I have a big breast. Maybe this should be cut off too." I told him that I saw nothing unusual, but I could not calm him down. He said he had developed ideas lately of wanting to be like the female patients. He wanted to be a woman, as his aunt had always wished him to be. He said that he was feeling unusually thirsty lately and was wondering whether he had diabetes. When I pointed out that he knew that his female friend on the ward was a diabetic, he agreed and hesitantly said that he was trying to be like her. "When I like people I try to imitate them and I want to be liked by them. I want people to say that I'm a nice guy. I'm trying to develop a good-natured personality, but then suddenly I hear a voice saying, 'You are no good. Hang yourself,' and then my spirits go down in the dumps." He said that he had not wanted to come to see me this morning, that he had hoped that I wouldn't get into one of these disturbing conversations with him. He added, "I'm hesitant. I know I want to face my problems but it's tough. It's like going to the electric chair, yet I know I have to do it. At such times I think of the girls and I say to myself, 'They like me. I'm wanted. I love it. I can't have enough of it.' But I don't like it when I start thinking that I'm turning into a woman. I don't like such thoughts. When I think this way I become afraid of the women patients. I feel inferior to them, and I have a bloated belly."

At the end of the interview, I reassured him as well as I could and promised to clear up with the head nurse any misunderstandings that might have arisen regarding his medication. He said that, as soon as I mentioned the name of the head nurse, two people had come to his mind, his aunt and his first girlfriend: "And they both should be dead. I want them dead because they will kill me." He also thought of the patient, Mrs. N., who had not returned to pay him a visit.

As the next two weeks went by, his passive and feminine wishes, as well as his tendency to become more dependent on me, grew more pronounced, and I heard less and less about his sexual interest for the women on the ward. During this period Tom had full control of his medication. I had also told him that he could decide about the length of the time of each interview. Sometimes the interviews lasted for a few minutes, at other times for several hours. He also asked to be allowed to see me two or three times a day, but generally he did not abuse these privileges.

A few days later Tom talked to me about going away to visit his family for the weekend. When I raised the problem of medication, he said he expected that "our plan" should be applied to the weekend visit. I replied that I did not think this could be done, since our plan applied only to the hospital ward. I suggested that he think it over and then present to me a detailed account of the drugs he felt he would need to take along with him during the two-day visit. He was upset at first, but grudgingly decided to give in because, he said, he realized there was some logic in what I said after all.

Two hours later he asked to see me and handed me a list. On it appeared the names of the drugs he was receiving daily on the ward. I said that the request seemed reasonable to me, but I reminded him that he was receiving demerol by injection. I suggested his taking the same amount by mouth which, of course, would not be as strong. He accepted this and started to make preparations for his weekend. He spoke at length about his expectations and felt he would be able to achieve a great deal. He appreciated my confidence in him, which, he claimed, had given him strength, and he said he was going to show me that he was worthy of my trust. He added that it would be difficult to be away from the hospital, where he felt he was now respected; at the same time, he recognized that he needed his independence very much.

Tom left the ward after shaking hands with all the patients and the nurses and after giving me a solemn promise that he was going to conduct himself well while away from the hospital.

He returned two days later in good spirits. He triumphantly produced two small bottles of pills, saying he had used only one fourth of the amount he had been given. He said he had had a very good time and had suffered little pain, so he had not needed as much medication. He apparently wanted to show me how good he had been, and he acted as if he were presenting me with a gift by returning three fourths of the pills. I was pleased, indeed, by this development, because I hoped that Tom was starting to control his drug addiction. At the same time I was puzzled by the fact that someone who had been on heavy doses of demerol, barbiturates, and codeine was able for two entire days to take only one fourth of the total amount of drugs he had been receiving in the hospital. Still, whatever hopes I had were premature.

The next day Tom complained that he had had a rough night and that he felt tired and weak. He said he was surprised, because he had done so well over the weekend. He assured me that he had tried all that day to remain on the amount of medication he had taken on the weekend, but was unable to do so. In two days he was back to his old formula, and all the gains had been wiped out. The reason he gave for this was that the nurses would always find excuses not to give him what he requested and that this attitude infuriated him. In a way he was right. As mentioned before, I had kept the nurses informed about the details of the treatment and had urged them to give freely whatever Tom requested. But changes of this type are not made overnight when they go against a long teaching tradition that nurses should never allow patients to handle narcotics. Also, I was aware that many of the nurses felt antagonistic toward the patient, although on the surface they appeared to accept his treatment. The head nurse on one occasion raised with me the question of the ultimate responsibility for our actions, since they defied every nursing principle and dogma she knew of. I reminded her that there were no nursing dogmas, only traditions, and reassured her that the responsibility was mine alone since I was the one who prescribed the medications. Despite all this, I found it difficult to convince her. She was a young and somewhat rigid person who liked only "routine." In contrast, Tom had an easier time with the night supervisor, who was sympathetic and easygoing. He had emphasized to me that his difficulties occurred usually during the day, and he attributed this to the lack of understanding on the part of the day head nurse. But he admitted that he also liked to complain to me about her.

In his interviews Tom continued to talk about his pain and to describe at length his fantasies about his anatomy. On one occasion I asked him to draw pictures of what he thought his insides looked like. He drew a bizarre picture of himself with a big mouth and with a long tubelike body. It possessed both male and female genitals. He described his pain as "the punch that I would like to throw against people whom I want to strike and destroy."

DOCTOR: Whom do you have in mind?
TOM: The head nurse for one. Mostly women come to mind.
DOCTOR: Anyone else?
TOM: Well, the thought I just had was about my aunt.

She spanked me because I used to wet the bed until I was eleven years old.

DOCTOR: I didn't know it lasted for so long.

TOM: Yes. I never mentioned this to the other doctors either. I was ashamed of it, I guess. It's funny because I told them about everything else. Well, anyway, my aunt used to rub my nose on the wet mattress. She used to threaten to put the bed in the cellar and get some rats in it to eat me up. I was terrified. I thought that the rats would tear me to pieces with their sharp teeth. I always tried so hard to please her, but deep inside I hated her. I felt left out and lonely. I had no one to turn to. My uncle used to beat me all the time, but somehow I preferred being beaten because it was out in the open. My aunt was sneaky. Both she and my uncle used to dress me in girls' clothes.

DOCTOR: Yes, I know.

TOM: Well, the funny thing is that at times I didn't mind it so much. I never admitted this before. It was some kind of a protection, but other times I hated them for humiliating me so. I worked like a dog, dying to show them I was good enough, but they didn't care. My fingers are crooked from the hard work. Later on when my uncle lost his job and we had nothing to eat, I supported them. As you know, after a while my uncle accepted me as an equal, but my aunt never liked me. She hated me to the very end. Even now that she is dead I still hate her. But you can't punish dead people.

DOCTOR: So you punish yourself?

He was taken aback by this question and said he wanted to die though he realized how illogical such a thought might be to others. But he added that ever since he had awakened from the operation he had felt he was going to die; the pain was a constant reminder of this.

After a routine visit by the surgeon, the patient asked to

see me and appeared angry. He claimed that the doctor had told him that his infection was chronic and could not be cured. This statement had particularly annoyed him because he was reminded of his own ideas of suicide and of killing others. "Sometimes I have an urge, almost a temptation, to push people around." He remembered once getting into a fight with two other men and having the urge to kill them then, but he did nothing but stare at them. They ignored him and soon left. He had the fantasy that they had read his mind and knew that he was going to kill them because he hated them. He remembered a similar episode, when he was working at the shipyards, at which time he was ready to push a man into the ocean and was so frightened that he did not dare move. Following this interview Tom asked for extra medication. When I saw him later that day, he said that our interview in the morning had bothered him and he had felt anxious ever since then. I tried to find out what specifically had bothered him, but he resisted:

TOM: I don't remember anything about it. My mind is completely blank. There is a block—some kind of a wall that cuts all the scenery out. I can't see. I don't remember. Everything is confused. I can't figure out anything. I'm in a fog. I ask for medication and I get mad. The pain gets worse. I kick a chair and I break it. I try to relax and I get mad. I'm going to smash everything. Then I think of you.

DOCTOR: Why are you angry at me?

TOM: I fought the thing off but I couldn't prevent it. I thought of you controlling the medication when you first took over. I picked up the flowerpot and I wanted to smash it against the window, but I told myself not to do it. I waited a while but then, bang, I broke it. The nurses got upset. I went into my room and took some medication to quiet down but I couldn't get rid of my anger. The other day you asked me if I wanted another operation so as to stay in the hospital and be taken care of. That's the last thing I want. I definitely do not want any more operations. That's all I can handle right now.

He seemed to be getting more and more upset: "What should I do? You are at fault." I answered that I understood how he felt and asked him to talk about his angry feelings for me. He continued, "I wanted to smash everything to bits—the lightbulb, the plates, the furniture in the room, and then there was that flowerpot. Your name was written all over it." He continued to talk in this way for some time. Despite the outburst, I was not convinced that Tom was as angry as he pretended to be.

DOCTOR: I'm glad you can express your anger at me so directly, but I have the impression that you're not as angry as you sound.

TOM: I'm very mad at you, but it's not like it used to be when you took over. Then I could really hate you, now I'm angry, but at the same time I think of all the things you have done for me, and it takes the edge off my rage.

By the end of the interview he seemed a little more relaxed. The next day he described an episode in which he had asked for medication, had to wait for twenty minutes, and during that time had lost the urge for it. "I can't get over the medication business, Doc. I'm mad at the nurses. You order something for me and it's mine. But they won't give it to me—they don't give me something that's mine. They take it away from me. They tear it away from me. I had the thought while I was waiting that my whole back-side was taken away from me. It was all gone, torn away from me. They cut it out of me, threw it out and broke it." He again seemed to be getting angry and confused. "I wanted to have a drink. It had a special meaning, but they wouldn't give it to me. I had to wait. The drink was for a celebration. My friend was going to come and visit me, and we could drink together. You know something, I think that when they refuse my medication they also hurt you because I know how much you care for me, cold as you may be. I deeply believe that you're really hurt—that you really care. But the nurses take it away from me, and smash it to bits." Such ups and downs occurred in his interviews quite regularly from this point on.

As time went by and Tom became more depressed and isolated, his demands increased. He started to eat a great deal. He was insatiable.

TOM: My appetite is ferocious. I crave for all kinds of foods. I had a dream last night. I was all dressed up in my best clothes, walking up and down the street. It was a street I have never seen before, lined up with beautiful houses and lovely fruit trees all in bloom. The colors were so vivid that I can still see them. I entered one of these houses. It was a real palace with marble stairs. It had a huge dining room, but there were no people, no one to be seen. In the middle there was a huge table full of all kinds of sea food, shrimps, lobsters, clams, as well as pies, cakes, candies of all sorts. I sat down and started to eat, but everything I touched made me feel sick to my stomach. I remember saying, "No food, no life." That was the end of the dream.

DOCTOR: What associations do you have?

TOM: Eating all by oneself is no fun at all. You might as well eat grass. But it makes me mad not to be able to enjoy things. I'm used to this kind of a torture, Doc. There is

never any happiness or enjoyment, and when finally I get
what I desire it backfires on me.

He asked for extravagant foods. On one occasion he asked
me if he might have imported lobster meat because his
uncle had once talked about it. When I said he could have
whatever he wanted, he asked for more and more, finally
in one day consuming ten cans of imported lobster. This
resulted in a stomach upset by the end of the day; but the
next day he wanted to offer lobster to all the other patients,
and, despite the objections of the dietitians who doubted
the therapeutic aspects of such a venture, Tom got permission to have a party and serve lobster to all the other patients
on the ward. Needless to say, they appreciated it. Starting
then, he went on an eating binge. He consumed lobster,
roast beef, steak, chicken, all kinds of fancy foods. (The
patient's bill was paid by a special grant, and so we were
able to meet the added expenses.)

As Tom's demands for medication increased, the hostility
of some of the nurses also increased. When the patient was
presented to the staff conference, the head nurse described
the treatment as "silly" and the patient's demands as extravagant. I was impressed by her antagonism to the patient and
suspected that she was somewhat jealous of all the attention
Tom was receiving, as well as of all the special privileges he
had. Her statements, however, led to considerable criticism
of the treatment by several staff members.

A special conference was called by the chief of service,
and I presented to the psychiatry staff the problems that I
had encountered in treating Tom and the reasons why my
supervisor and I had decided to try the anaclitic treatment.
The head nurse was then asked to express her opinions, and
she presented an unexpectedly objective picture of what

was going on. To my surprise, however, one of the doctors spoke about a patient he was treating who was jealous of Tom, and then he strongly criticized the unrealistic aspects of the anaclitic therapy. Following this, a staff doctor got up and ridiculed our experiment. It was preposterous to give in to an addict and offer him narcotics, and it was foolishness, he said, to feed the patient expensive and extravagant foods. He thought that our whole department was becoming the laughing stock of the hospital, and advised me to learn first of all the accepted ways of treating patients before embarking on wild experimentation. Society, he reminded me, took a dim view of such novel procedures. All this resulted in a temporary order from the chief of service to discontinue the anaclitic treatment.

At first I felt very disappointed after the conference. I went to see Tom to announce the news to him. He had known about the meeting and was waiting in his room eagerly for my arrival, but he immediately sensed what had happened.

TOM: So it didn't go so well.

DOCTOR: The treatment is off, Tom. No foods. No free drugs. We must go back to the old regime.

TOM: You look very sad, Doc. Cheer up. What did you expect?

DOCTOR: I certainly didn't expect so much hostility for trying to do something new.

TOM: You are young and inexperienced. It is an extravagant treatment and, furthermore, it makes people jealous. People are afraid of novelty. Don't worry about it. I'll do all I can to help you out.

I thanked Tom for his understanding: the roles had been reversed and the patient was treating the doctor.

All that day I could not stop thinking about what the staff had said during the conference. The words "society takes a dim view," "the laughing stock of the hospital," "the accepted ways," kept going through my mind. Why is there always this need for conformity? Why is originality so frightening? I remembered a conversation I had had in occupied Paris during World War II with a German soldier. He said that I was naive to believe that there was a chance of Germany's losing the war. It was absolutely inconceivable to him. The trouble with people like me was that we did not accept facts. The new order in Europe, he said, was a fait accompli, and it was the duty of everybody to accept it. He said that he had an argument with a doctor friend of his who had been drafted into the army in the early days of the Hitler regime, because this friend wanted to be a doctor first, a soldier second, and refused to see the accepted way of doing things. Later on, however, the doctor had changed his mind and even became a member of the SS. With much vehemence the German soldier emphasized that his friend had signed on the "dotted line." I had remembered this encounter after the end of the war, when I read about the obedience of some German doctors to the Nazi party, their acceptance of this fait accompli. They were the ones who without protest performed horrible crimes on their suffering patients. Did the staff doctors view my experiment as a similar crime? Was it only Hitler's society that took a dim view of anyone who could think independently and who dared challenge it? I thought I knew the answer.

I soon realized that my disappointment had turned into anger. I thought of Tom's words, "What did you expect?" and "People are afraid of novelty." Kafka's *Trial* came to my mind. K. was horrified when he realized that "everybody belonged to the Court." His only crime was that he did not belong—his fate was sealed in advance. He had "to die like a dog." The same thing happened to Meursault in *The Stranger*. His crime was not that he had killed an Arab; this could be easily forgiven. Camus makes it clear that his real crime had to do with his bizarre behavior and his independent life, which had challenged society. This could not be forgiven, and he also had to die. These thoughts convinced me that I should take action. I decided to talk to my chief first thing in the morning. The next day I saw the chief of service and explained the reasons why I thought the anaclitic treatment should continue. I emphasized that, although it was new and possibly extravagant, it seemed to be the last resort, and it had already produced a basic change for the better in the patient-doctor relationship. He listened attentively, and after a few minutes of silence said that he had reconsidered. He gave me permission to resume.

Jubilant, I went to see Tom.

TOM: So we can go ahead [smiling].

DOCTOR: You read me like an open book, Tom.

TOM: Yes, I know! It's written all over your face.

DOCTOR: I'm very happy. The chief gave me permission to go ahead. You helped me a great deal by what you said yesterday. I want to thank you.

TOM: Forget it, Doc.

DOCTOR: I'm really grateful to you. I did a lot of thinking last night. One must learn to compromise with society and to live according to the rules, but always there should be a way out. One should sign the contract only if there is a clause for independent action.

TOM: I'm glad to see you happy.

DOCTOR: Thank you very much.

CHAPTER VIII

ADDICTION

DESPITE his voracious appetite, Tom remained depressed. Several times we switched round from demerol to codeine and back again. In his interviews he talked about being fed up with life. He told me the story of a man who thought he had discovered some money, and when it turned out to be toy money he wanted to kill himself. Tom said he had also met nice people in his life, but they all had abandoned him—his girlfriends, his old woman friend, Mrs. N., his family—so suicide was the only answer. "I cannot separate myself from the person I like. I feel that we are the same person, we share the same body, the same life. When you take us apart, there's a big black hole that is left in one of the two. I am the one with the big black hole and I have one here to prove it." He pointed at the ileostomy and started to cry. Later on he complained that he was unable to sleep, because of a repetitious dream about a big "black pit."

As the next two weeks passed. Tom became more and more preoccupied with himself until his self-centeredness was extremely pronounced. Every phrase would start with an "I." He had lost interest in the "treatment of the other patients." He talked about himself in derogatory terms, calling himself "an old bushel basket, a bag of death." He said he wanted to cut off his head and offer it to me. Slowly he started taking more demerol, until he had increased it to a daily nineteen injections of 50 mg. each. This was the largest amount he had used up to that time. In the interviews he talked about his aunt more and more often—her vicious-ness, her hot temper, and her coldness. These qualities reminded him of the head nurse. He also remembered with anger how his mother had liked his brother better. He started to think about masturbation and associated this with mas-turbating when he was a child and feeling very guilty about it. He remembered that he was afraid to talk to girls be-cause he masturbated and he knew it was wrong. Ever since, whenever he lay in bed, he would always think of himself as a child and remember about lying down in bed and masturbating, and being afraid he would be caught by his uncle or aunt. But it was always his aunt who would catch him and punish him. He talked about his aunt's lack of affection, his need for affection, how he always had had the feeling of being alone, and how he could never tolerate the thought of his aunt and his uncle together. "I was always alone; no one ever hugged me." He described his aunt as unattractive, undesirable, and disgusting. He said he was unable to understand what his uncle could find in her and furthermore, "She never gave anything to anyone."

TOM: When I think of her my pain gets always worse, and then as I think of the pain I forget about the bad thoughts. Now my incision, for instance, hurt a great deal last night. I wanted to rip it open.

DOCTOR: Was it the incision or some person you wanted to rip open?

TOM: There you are! I knew who it was all along but I just turned it against myself, as you've pointed out so often. Last night I felt very lonely. I asked for medication, but it didn't help, so you know what I did, I knelt next to my bed and I prayed. I don't know the God I was praying to, but I did pray. Later on I felt like crying.

DOCTOR: What were you praying for?

TOM: I was praying for forgiveness for all the nasty, dirty, vile things that I have thought of . . .

He started to cry and left the office. I followed him to his room and tried to soothe him, but he said that he wanted to be alone. After a while, the head nurse mentioned that he had asked to see me. I found him lying on his bed, moaning.

TOM: I try and try to ignore the voices, but I've been hearing echoes since yesterday. Now you know why I ran out of your office. I heard her voice, "You are doomed," she said. "You must die." She kept on repeating the same thing over and over.

DOCTOR: Why didn't you want to talk about it?

TOM: I don't know. I talked about these voices before, but yesterday I got scared. I felt sick inside—discouraged. I just want to give up. I felt sorry for myself. The medications don't hold me any more. I know I've been getting extra ones lately.

DOCTOR: I know, but there were other times when you asked for more medication, and after a while you decreased the amount all by yourself.

TOM: Yes, but it's getting harder and harder. I'm all mixed up. I feel proud and I feel guilty at the same time. I sleep and I wake up. I eat a lot and then I have no appetite. I feel close to you, yet other times I'm mad at you. I hate to ask for medication. I hate to ask you to increase it, but this is what I want you to do.

DOCTOR: You know you can have all you want.

TOM: Yes, but maybe I should be getting a higher dose every time. I tried to get hold of you three times yesterday, but they told me you were busy. The last time they said you were gone. It made me feel sad—as though there were no one to care for me. I was all alone in the world.

DOCTOR: You were angry at me, and you turned the anger at yourself. You did the same thing when you were angry at your aunt.

TOM: Yes, I know, but it didn't help this time. I am a coward.

I tried to reassure him by emphasizing my continued interest in him, and by the end of the interview he seemed to be in better spirits. In the next few days I made a special effort to see him briefly two or three times a day, in addition to the time we spent in our regular interviews. His mood seemed to improve a little bit.

Throughout this time, despite being depressed and self-preoccupied, Tom still attempted to use his good mind to find a logical explanation for his condition. In his interviews he continued to reminisce about his experiences with his aunt and uncle. He always remembered the unpleasant experiences, such as his uncle kicking him in the back when he tried to ride on the sides of streetcars. He said that if his uncle did not find out about this, there would always be a policeman who would catch him, and he also would kick him in the back. He associated the stabbing pains in his back with these earlier experiences. He seemed to derive some pleasure in talking about these subjects, and when I pointed this out to him he said it was better to be kicked in the back than to be completely ignored.

In another interview he again started to discuss his wish to improve the ileostomy bag so that he would be of benefit to other people with similar problems. But he would soon return to his familiar request for more medication. During this time, he remained friendly to me, but there was also an underlying hostility. "You're the best of the three doctors I've had. You never refuse me anything. You make things easier for me. I think you're O.K., but you leave me no openings for resentment." When I suggested that maybe he resented this very fact, he agreed. "Maybe this is true, Doc. I hope that one day you're going to make a mistake and say 'No' to my request for medication so that I can really let you have it—blast you right out of the way." There was, however, a childlike quality in these outbursts. He said he hated having responsibilities and was glad when he realized that I had, in addition to him, more responsibilities on my shoulders because I had the whole world to worry about.

From the physical standpoint, a new complication appeared. The infection on the patient's abdomen started to spread until it involved his umbilical region, where several abscesses developed and discharged pus and serosanguineous material. His reaction to this was peculiar. He complained that the pain affected his sex organs—that he felt numb and was unable to masturbate any more, which made him mad because it was his only pleasure.

Tom came to me at this point and said that the day before he had had only fifteen shots of demerol, each 50 mg., but that he was worried because his appetite was not as good as it had been in the past. He said that every time he looked at food he started to have severe abdominal pain. "Just talking about food bothers me. There is something wrong with the food, although I know it's the best food in the world. I can't understand it. I don't eat now, and instead of losing weight I'm gaining. I should be feeling so much better, but I feel so much worse. I can't explain all this." He then somewhat dramatically announced that, for the second time in a month, he had heard voices and the voices were saying, "You must get out of here. You must die. Kill yourself, Tom. You must kill yourself."

TOM: I got frightened and for the first time I answered

them back. I said, "Why do you speak to me now? What have I done?" The voice answered, "You are no good; you must suffer. You must turn into a woman." I said, "Should I kill myself? Is this what you want? Can I find peace if I kill myself?" He answered ......

DOCTOR: So it was a man's voice.

TOM: Yes. I didn't recognize whose voice it was. It said, "No, you don't have to kill yourself because then you will kill me too, and you don't want to do that. You don't want to silence me. I am here to keep you company, Tom, because you are all alone." You see, Doc, it was true in a funny sort of a way. I was lonely. I thought of playing cards but there was no one to play with. You were very much in my mind. I wanted to be with you, to talk with you all night, but I didn't have the nerve to ask for you.

DOCTOR: So in a strange way the voices kept you company.

TOM: Yes, they did. It's the truth. I was scared but they did keep me company.

I was quite impressed by this dialogue between Tom and his voices. Unpleasant, frightening, and painful as they might have been, the hallucinations seemed to serve a purpose, in a bizarre way. They managed to alleviate my patient's loneliness. I asked him to talk more about the voices.

TOM: Well, you see when I was young, living with my aunt, there were times when my uncle would go on a binge. He would be away for a couple of days, even longer. During these times I was all alone with my aunt. I used to talk to her but she never answered. She was mad at my uncle but she wouldn't say a word to him when he came back. *Not a single word.* This would go on for weeks. But this didn't happen all the time. She also had a biting tongue and she could tell him off using every dirty word you ever heard of. He liked it better that way. He hated her silence and I hated it too. It was so lonely, not a sound in the house.

DOCTOR: Well, what about these voices now?

TOM: I don't know, but my loneliness now reminds me of the times when my aunt would be quiet. I used to pray for a human voice but it was no good. All was so silent. It was terrible.

DOCTOR: Did you hear voices when you were young?

TOM: No. I never heard a voice before all this trouble began.

DOCTOR: Well, then?

TOM: There is a feeling I have and it's hard to explain. When the voice started accusing me I was terrified, as I told you, but it was like the times when I was alone with my aunt. It was a dream come true. Of course, nothing happens the right way for me.

DOCTOR: You mean that the voices shouldn't have been accusing?

TOM: Yes. Why can't I hear voices that say sweet things to my ears? Why not hear Mrs. N.'s voice or someone else's, telling me they love me, they care for me, but I know it will never happen. I wish it would.

DOCTOR: Well, there are better ways. Company from real people is much superior to company from your voices, Tom.

TOM: Maybe you're right.

He again associated the voices with his operation. He remembered having the fantasy that the patient who was lying next to him while he was on the surgical floor was going to have an operation to be "de-sexed." "The thought occurred to me that this is what I wanted. If you have no sex, then you have no problems." He remembered the last time he had had sexual intercourse and how unsatisfactory it was. It had become an ordeal for him because he always was left with a feeling that he was being damaged. He remembered how the voices used to say, "Tom, you're a half-man. You look like hell." At such times he compulsively had to look at his body very carefully to see if there was anything wrong with him. "I looked all over my skin where I saw all the old scars from the transfusions and from the IV's and at my abdomen where I saw the scar from the operation, and at that ileostomy bag, and I was reminded that I am half a man and that the voices are right." When I asked why he felt he was a half-man, he said he could not understand his mixed feelings because, on the one hand, he wanted to be de-sexed and, on the other hand, he was afraid of it. He remembered that the first question he had asked the surgeon after the operation was whether his testicles had been cut off with a knife. Thoughts of this kind always made him feel mixed up. He also remembered that he had confused a woman patient with his aunt, and when he had had sexual feelings for this woman he thought this meant that he had sexual feelings for his aunt. He then added, "Why am I saying all this to you? It must be wrong—it must be. It doesn't apply to me, but the thought keeps recurring and I'm mad at you because you're a psychiatrist."

But Tom's communications during the interviews continued to be confused. He talked about deriving pleasure from his rectum as other people derived pleasure from their sexual organs. He remembered that when he had had constipation, before the onset of his ulcerative colitis, a bowel movement always gave him an erection and an emission at the same time. Following this disclosure he appeared anxious, and ten minutes after I had left him one of the nurses told me that he had asked to see me. I was eager to get the interview over with, because I had to discuss a paper at our psychiatry conference. Tom was aware of this, but insisted that he had to ask me a very special favor. In dramatic tones he told me that after having talked with me about the woman patient and his aunt, he had suddenly been reminded of his uncle. He said he thought there was a parallel between his uncle and me, and that this had all of a sudden become quite clear to him. He said, "I hated my uncle, but then I got to like him and from then on we became very close. It's the same thing with you, Doc. I hated you when I knew you were going to come over and take the place of my previous psychiatrist; but then I grew to respect you, particularly after you helped me out with the medication and showed how you could help me with my other problems. There is something big here and I feel I want to celebrate. This is a very important event that has a lot of meaning to me."

I realized that Tom was trying to communicate something unusual to me, but at the same time I was in a hurry to get to the staff conference. I felt ambivalent and did not know what to do, but Tom was not going to give up. "Doctor," he said, "we must have a drink together. Could we have a drink right now? I want two and a half ounces of whiskey for me and the same amount for you." I knew that this would be an exact repetition of the event with his uncle in the cellar when they signed "a declaration of peace," as the patient had called it, when he was thirteen years old. I decided to let him have the whiskey. It was eleven o'clock in the morning, and the last thing I wanted to do was to have a drink; but I accepted his offer, telling him I would take only a sip, and so we spent the next five minutes "celebrating." I felt that this event was a re-enactment that seemed to convince Tom, in a very realistic way, that I had accepted him, as his uncle had accepted him twenty years earlier.

It must be remembered that the patient's ulcerative colitis began soon after his uncle's death; and that we were attempting in the anaclitic treatment to convince him that he could trust people emotionally and to help him destroy the vicious idea that he would have to lose every person he trusted and loved. Before leaving him I told him that I was not going to abandon him. He smiled significantly.

He seemed better the next day—better than I had seen him for some weeks. He said that having that drink with me was evidence of my trusting him. In the afternoon of the same day, however, his mood changed. He again became depressed. He wrote me a note saying that he had thought of undertakers coming for him because he was rotten inside and that this was evidenced by the discharge from his umbilicus. Later on he came to show me the discharge: "It's all dead and rotten." Then he stopped suddenly; his face changed; he became pale and started to shake. He blurted out that he had the fantasy that his aunt was inside, deep inside his bowels, and he could not get rid of her because she was a "bitch." At this he became alarmed and seemed more and more confused. "She is inside me, eating me up, sucking at my insides, tearing them to pieces, eating my rotten blood, and I'm trying to get her out by vomiting." He talked rapidly and became even more upset. He said he was convinced that he was going out of his mind. My reassurings made no difference; he did not seem to listen and became increasingly disturbed. I told him that he had been fighting to understand these terrible feelings and that he was doing a valiant job, but I added that it had all come up suddenly after the interview of the previous day, when we had had a drink together. "I am a damn sick guy, Doc. I am very, very sick." At this point he asked me if he could go ahead and have drinks on the same free basis as his medications. I took him over to the head nurse's desk and told her that Tom was to have 2½ ounces of whiskey once a day when he requested it. He tried to smile, but instead he broke down and started to cry.

CHAPTER IX

ALCOHOLISM

TOM'S demands for alcohol soon became the most perplexing problem we had yet had to cope with. He had been a heavy drinker in the past, and we knew that by allowing him to drink at this time we would be contributing toward the further development of his self-destructive attitude. On the other hand, we felt that a refusal of his requests for alcohol would be contrary to the spirit of the anaclitic treatment. After some deliberation, we decided to give our consent to his having 2½ ounces of whiskey twice a day.

He immediately started to ask for more and more whiskey. He tried to manufacture convincing reasons for his demands, but it was perfectly clear to us that he was simply trying to drown his fears in alcohol. He also continued to ask for his usual 50 mg. of demerol, given subcutaneously on a p.r.n. basis. In addition, he was getting a high-protein diet, supplemented by vitamins, and 100 mg. of nembutal for sleep, 1 gram of chloral hydrate by mouth every four hours, 300,000 units of penicillin daily, as well as vitamin A and B ointment for the skin lesions close to his ileostomy. On some days he shifted from demerol to codeine, and then asked to be put back on demerol again. He averaged approximately seventeen injections of 50 mg. each of demerol, making a total of 850 mg. for a twenty-four-hour period. The 2½ ounces of whiskey, requested twice a day at first, was increased to three times that amount, thus further complicating the problem. I hesitated for a while about giving him more than 2½ ounces, but he was quick to detect my reluctance and accused me of having doubts, of not trusting him, and of being "tired of it all." The nurses also strongly disapproved of the alcohol. But it soon became clear to me that unless I changed my attitude toward Tom's demands, the anaclitic treatment was going to fail. I therefore decided to take the great step and offer him all the alcohol he wanted. He thanked me profusely, saying he knew I would change my mind, and he added, "Anyway, Doc, I eat a lot." This was true. He consumed enormous amounts of food—lobster, steak, roast beef, and all sorts of fine delicacies —and his hospital bill was becoming accordingly enormous.

Soon he started to "celebrate" certain anniversaries and asked for even more whiskey. He warned me not to attempt to stop him. He said he felt at times that I had taken away his manhood and that alcohol was going to help him recover it. "It's like the first drink I had with my uncle," he said. And then he added, "I remember that once my uncle took away my toy rifle and smashed it, saying, 'A man doesn't need guns to protect his manhood. The only thing to do is to work hard and this will prove he is a man.' " He talked about the medications as "working" and "not working" when he felt strong or weak. At times he voiced his old suspicion that he was receiving placebos, but it was not difficult to show him that he was getting exactly what he wanted.

At another time Tom came in and announced to me that he knew the pain came from his inability to accept the fact that he had lost his rectum. "It was a painful rectum but it was there. Now I don't have anything but the pain." He then described his feelings after his second operation, when his rectum was removed. "I thought they made a mistake and they cut off a part of me. It was not in the bargain. They were going to cripple me—cause me pain. How long can I live like that? How much more can I stand? It's a hard job. It's at times like this that I want to punch someone—to strike—to hit—to kill. But I manage to do it on myself. Before the operation I used to punch my rectum because it meant death to me. And I still want to do it. I wanted to get rid of the rectum. I should have kept it, because keeping it would have meant being killed and I would be better off." He seemed to be depressed at the end of this interview. Later on, the nurses told me that the patient wanted to see me again. I entered his room and he greeted me with the following remarks:

TOM: I'm mad because I'm scared. It's a vague feeling but I'm going downhill, Doc, and I'm getting very, very mad.

DOCTOR: You're getting angry. Why?

TOM: I want to kill myself. What kind of life is this? All full of hate, fear, and pain. Full of people who think of themselves. No one cares about me. I have decided it's better to take action. I can do something about it. Thank goodness there's death!

DOCTOR: You're too confused to be thinking about making such an important decision as whether to live or to die.

TOM: But my life is my own. No one owns it except myself. I can do what I want with it.

DOCTOR: Tom, in a way you're right. The decision about one's own life is in his own hands and no one else's. I don't dispute that. What I say is that you are too confused from all this pain to think clearly about such an important subject.

TOM: You sound like a priest, Doc. I remember a priest who once told me that it was a sin to commit suicide. "The church is against all those who kill themselves," he said. I remember when I was arguing with him he told me that society could not exist if all the people had the right to kill themselves. There would be no society and no church. Is that what you believe?

DOCTOR: It's not a matter of belief. I think man's greatest

freedom is to be master of himself, master of his thoughts and his feelings. He has the right to decide whether he should live or die. Some of the greatest acts of heroism, in defiance to oppression, involve a decision about life under tyranny or freedom by a heroic death. To arrive at such an important decision, however, one must be thinking clearly at the time. His mind must be lucid. You cannot decide about death, Tom, because you're not thinking coherently, and therefore we must and will protect you from yourself.

TOM: I guess you're right, Doc, because deep inside I don't want to die. But I am scared and at times like this I don't know what to do.

DOCTOR: It seems to me, then, that we must try to understand what this fear is all about.

Tom seemed to be reassured, and for the next few days he appeared somewhat more relaxed.

During this period the ileostomy took on a particular meaning of strength and masculinity for the patient. He became terrified at the notion that it might become infected and "rot away," and that this would kill a part of himself. But, as with all such fantasies, he enjoyed the thought.

Following each interview, Tom would feel apprehensive and ask to see me again in an hour or two. He would then invariably complain of pain and talk about fear of accidents, his wishes to kill himself, and the hate that filled his mind. "Whiskey is the only way to chase such thoughts out of my mind," he said. He told me this was the real reason for his drinking and that he had to think up excuses when he told the nurses he was drinking to celebrate an anniversary.

Two weeks later, the patient started again to have a bloody discharge from the anal region, and the infection that had been well localized around his ileostomy began to spread until it involved the entire lower abdomen. The staphylococci that were responsible for the infection seemed to have developed a resistance to penicillin. As the infection grew worse, Tom became more and more depressed. During this phase the most striking feature was the sudden change in his eating habits. His appetite decreased and his requests for special foods stopped. One day he dramatically produced sixteen 100 mg. of nembutal capsules. He said he had collected them throughout his hospitalization with the thought that, if he were convinced that he could not get well, he was going to commit suicide. But he gave the capsules to me because he said he had felt depressed the previous night and was on the verge of taking them.

TOM: I had been thinking that if I attempted to kill myself people would be sorry for me and would not leave me. This way I could get what I wanted from them; I could be strong again. They would be my slaves. I would have full control over everybody, even over you, Doc. One of the patients told me that she had tried to kill herself just to scare her husband who had threatened to leave her for another woman. She succeeded, Doc, because her husband never left her from then on. He was scared to have her death on his conscience. She even tried to frighten her own psychiatrist with her threats of suicide. I was thinking the same way last night. I thought I might take a few pills and leave you a note saying that everyone who left me was to blame for my death, but I knew I couldn't do it. It would be no use because no one would believe it.

DOCTOR: I do believe you, Tom. I know you suffer a great deal. I know you're lonely. Suicide is not going to convince me further that you're unhappy.

TOM: I know all this, Doc, but I had the thought that if I killed myself everyone would gather in my room. The head nurse would call all the patients, the nurses, and the doctors, and then she would call you. You would come in and say, "Tom was the best patient I've ever had." I know it's all nonsense, but the urge was very great.

DOCTOR: I see what you mean, but I disagree with you. Don't forget your life is your own and no one else's.

I thanked him for returning the pills and tried to reassure him, but he continued to talk about his loneliness and the feeling that everybody had abandoned him, including his old friend, his brother, and his mother. He said all was rapidly coming to an end; he expressed much hatred for everyone, most of all for himself. But it was of significance to me that he expressed a feeling of going through a new phase in his treatment, one which he could not understand.

The next day he asked for and received twenty-two injections of demerol—a total of 1100 mg.—the largest amount he had ever received on a twenty-four-hour basis during his entire hospitalization. In addition, he had 2½ ounces of whiskey three times. He appeared to be withdrawn and said that he was rotten and that everything was a mess.

During one of our interviews, Tom talked a great deal about the woman patient, Mrs. N.

TOM: I found a gold mine in Mrs. N. and I can't have her because she is gone. Do you remember my telling you a story about a man who found a diamond mine but it turned out to be only glass and crystals, so he blew his brains out? All night long I've been thinking of Mrs. N. I cannot give her up. She has all her life ahead of her. But when I think of her, I think that she liked me and no one can tell me any different. I have to put her on a pedestal. It was so good to talk with her the way we used to. Last night I was just thinking about her and had no appetite. I only got one and a half hours of sleep. And you know something, Doc, she wanted a baby and I couldn't give her one. I wanted to cut off my head and offer it to her, but it's not worth very much. Do you understand any of this, Doc?

DOCTOR: Yes, I think I do.

TOM: It's hard for me to tell you all this. I can talk about the pain, about the nurses, about the food, but it's different when I start thinking about Mrs. N.

DOCTOR: Are you worried about my reaction?

TOM: That's not it, but I can't put my finger on ...... I try to think of the pain ...... I heard some voices ...... I want to say something ...... I don't know what it is ...... I want to get out of here. I don't want to die!

DOCTOR: I won't hurt you, Tom. Just tell me what comes to your mind.

TOM: Well ...... I'll tell you. You are good to me but I'm worried that I'm too much for you. You work too hard. I hope nothing happens to you. You never refuse me anything. You made things easier for me ...... I have so much pain ...... You are a good man. You leave me no openings for my resentment.

DOCTOR: I see.

TOM: Deep inside I hoped that you would say no when I asked for extra medication.

DOCTOR: In that way you can be angry at me, and you can give up the responsibility which is now in your hands?

TOM: No, not the responsibility. I figure you take a hell of a lot of responsibility on your shoulders, but I do want to be angry at you. I still have a discharge from my navel. I want to tell you about it. I am infected all over and the pain drives me whacky. It affects my sex organs.

DOCTOR: Are you worried about it?

TOM: After the operation I worried because I had no sexual drive. I thought I was impotent. I felt damaged. Look at this discharge now. I am not a man any more.

DOCTOR: You haven't told me why you are angry at me.

TOM: You asked for it, Doc. God damn it! You're asking too much. If you try to stop me ......

DOCTOR: What, Tom?

TOM: Mind your own business. You're trying to stop my feelings for Mrs. N.

At this point he started to cry and soon after got up and left.

The next day, Tom recalled that whenever Mrs. N. had complained about her ailments he would soon develop the same symptoms. He recalled that these identifications made sense to him because he felt that he was partly a woman. That same afternoon one of his abscesses discharged pus and blood. Tom seemed to be upset when I saw him. He opened up his bathrobe and showed me his umbilicus, which seemed to be discharging pus.

TOM: I want to tell you about my belly button. I have an infection in there and the pain drives me mad. The pain also affects my sex organs. When I get a shot of penicillin I get a discharge from my penis. Am I imagining all this? A patient once told me that during an operation it is possible to have the doctors de-sex you. I'm worried. Maybe they did this to me. Maybe they made a mistake and I don't know about it. Last time I had intercourse it was not satisfactory. It left me with a bad feeling. I say to myself, maybe you are damaged as hell. Yesterday I heard some voices coming from the TV set, "You're a half-man, Tom. You look like hell." I wanted to throw something at the TV screen. When a patient asked me what the matter was, I didn't answer. I thought the surgeons may have cut something out. Last night I had a fantasy I was carrying a baby down there. [He pointed to his abdomen.] What is this discharge from my navel, Doc? Maybe it has to do with this baby. I can't give Mrs. N. a baby so I'm carrying a baby for her ......

DOCTOR: How long have you had the fantasy of being a pregnant woman?

TOM: I remember carrying my aunt inside my bowel before the surgeons cut it off. She was eating me up, from the inside, that's why I had all this blood when I had diarrhea. Sure I'm a woman, Doc. If you're a woman you're better off.

DOCTOR: Whom are you married to then?

TOM: To my old man and now to you. [He sighed, then blurted out:] I am a damned sick guy. I feel sick. These double feelings. I'm carrying a baby. I have pain. I'm a woman. It's all so mixed up.

DOCTOR: It's our job to separate the reality from the fantasy, and I think we can do it.

Tom seemed to be restless and I realized that he wanted to leave so I stopped the interview. The next day he avoided me, and when I confronted him with this he admitted that he did not want to talk to me.

DOCTOR: Why are you afraid of me?

TOM: I don't know. I'm upset today. I need whiskey badly ...... Something came to my mind last night. I don't remember ...... [He looked very upset.] Let me go, Doc.

DOCTOR: You can go if you want to, Tom.

TOM: Well, here it is ...... [He produced a towel stained with blood and put it on the desk.] You wanted the evidence—here it is. Menstruation—pains and bloody kotex—it all ties together. I am a woman who is showing off, who exhibits herself to show to everybody that she is a female.

[He started to laugh and continued to laugh for a long time.] I've got to be the woman I guess. I'll rot. [He started to mumble something about pain.]

DOCTOR: How is your pain today?

TOM: Comes and goes. [He was silent for a long time.] It's thoughts of this kind that are responsible for my getting so many needles. I'm getting to be a pincushion. What does it mean? I need all these needles to prove I'm a woman. I'm confused. Nothing makes sense. I don't want to have such thoughts. I want to keep them out of my mind—to swallow them. I used to swallow some thoughts and they would come out like blood in my stools. They would eat my insides and tear them to bits, but now I have no bowels, so they will stay in me and kill me. I feel so weak, like a helpless little bag.

He was silent for a long time and then, with tremendous anger, said, "I want to swallow her up—to become a part of her—to be half-woman and half-man." He struggled to his feet and left the office. Later on that day Tom became belligerent and profane on the ward, and was asked by the nurses to go to the closed ward during the night.

His appearance changed very rapidly. He looked sad and his face was pale and drawn; his demands for medication increased and he drank a great deal; and he asked constantly to see me. We had anticipated that as the patient regressed he would ask more from me in terms of frequent visits and emotional support, but I was apprehensive, fearing I would be unable to satisfy all his demands and strong dependent needs. When I went to visit him later that day, I found him crying in his room. He told me that every time he had thought of food that day, even of refreshments, he would have severe pains, and he could not eat anything because he felt like vomiting. He said he thought of food or drink as poison—swallowing it was going to kill him. I pointed out to him that he had had similar fears before and had found them to be only fantasies, but I was unable to calm him down. When I asked if there was anything specific that frightened him, he answered that he had recently felt more afraid of me, but he was unable to explain just what was happening to him. He repeated the same complaints of feeling depressed and of knowing he was going to die, like all the people whom he had loved—his father, uncle, and grandmother. "As they left me I felt as if I had inside me a big black hole. I felt that I was going to join them soon. I loved S. [this was his old friend] and she is also going to die. I don't believe in anything any more. I loved my grandmother and I had to bury my love in her coffin." He associated this to his wanting to jump inside his grandmother's grave and continued, "I eat, I don't; I vomit, I don't; I let everything go. Last night and this morning I have pains in my groin. I thought I was going crazy. I got some whiskey and tried to drown my feelings, but it didn't help. My hands felt weak. Food, whiskey, pain—it's all the same." He flushed and looked very tense. "I just suddenly thought that I want to swallow you," he blurted out. "This means I want to kill you, Doctor. Everything that goes inside me means killing." He remained agitated after this, and later on during the night he asked to see me again. The auditory hallucinations had become more threatening. The voices were accusing him, calling him "dirty names," insulting him. I thanked him for revealing all this to me, and he asked to be transferred to the closed ward for protection. He continued to express anger at everyone around him that night. "Nobody brings me anything to eat, even if I am going to throw it up. They all want me to die. I don't know what's going

on. I'm discharging pus through my belly button; I carry
bloody towels. I feel I have nowhere to go to, nothing to do.
Why? Why?"

DOCTOR: Maybe ......

TOM: Don't lie to me, Doc, like everybody else. I don't
care anymore. I don't think I'll get better anyway. No need
for it. Everybody has died. Everything is futile. I made up
my mind not to get better. What's the use? For whom?

DOCTOR: Yourself.

TOM: I'll be God-damned alone.

DOCTOR: No, Tom.

TOM: Oh yes, Doc, and you know it. I talk like a pregnant
woman. I'm all puffed up. I'm losing weight. I'm not eating.
My belly button is getting bigger and bigger. I'm carrying
a baby. It's not Mrs. N.'s baby. I don't want to see her when
she comes to visit next Tuesday because I won't give her
the gift that she's praying for. The baby is a bastard! We
have to name it after you. It doesn't sound so bad, does it?
It must be yours. It's so funny.

He was silent and then he started to shake. He became
visibly pale, tried to stand up, and fainted.

The next day the nurses told me that Tom had taken
only eleven 50 mg. injections of demerol and no whiskey.
For the next four days he abstained from drinking, but he
appeared to be more depressed. He told me he had given up
hope and was convinced that he was going to die. "I don't
know what's going on. Even the whiskey doesn't help any
more, so I gave it up. I am discharging pus through my
belly button. Blood comes out of my anus. Everything is
falling apart. I'm breaking up into pieces. What I see in
front of me is a big black pit. It is a big black hole that I'm
headed for and I'm scared, Doc, because I don't know what

it's all about." He said that this feeling had been growing stronger for the last ten days and was the reason for his refusing to eat and his wanting to kill himself. "Why do I have to face this black pit, Doctor? It scares me so, and then it brings up a terrific rage in me. I have destroyed everyone and everything around me and there is only one way to get out of this fear—the best way out—the best way I know, and that is to kill myself." I was convinced that Tom was so afraid to see what was in this black pit that he preferred to destroy himself. I asked myself, "What is he trying to say? What is it that he wants? What is this pit?"

The next day he appeared better. He said that everything had become clear to him the night before. "I suddenly realized that at first I wanted to be independent, to get well, to stand on my own two feet and to go back to work, but now that I have been completely abandoned by everybody I feel that I don't want to go on and that the best thing for me is to die." I tried to point out to him that this would be no solution. Hoping for death was only an indefinite postponement of his problems, like drawing a curtain in front of a window so as not to see what is on the other side of it. I said, "You have a peculiar notion that you are able to kill people, but this is only a frightening idea—a fantasy in your mind. You have not killed anyone. All these ideas of yours have nothing to do with reality." I realized later how futile all this was—to try to control with mere words these overwhelming emotional feelings that Tom was expressing. It was even paradoxical that I was attempting to emphasize reality when at the same time I was helping the patient to regress.

Tom, in the meanwhile, continued to be depressed. He said that he knew he was working against himself and against our common efforts, but admitted there was pleasure in being able to defeat himself. Later on that same day he wanted to see me again. He complained of feeling miserable and talked about how everyone was letting him down. When I asked him if he thought that I also was letting him down, he admitted that he wasn't sure, but that the thought had occurred to him. Again he said that he had only one alternative because he was caught between the devil and the deep black pit. The devil was his rage, he said. How could anyone want to live, wanting to hurt everybody? "How can I be so cruel? The voices accuse me all the time. Nothing makes sense to me." He suddenly started to laugh and then burst into tears. After a while he quieted down and said, in a hesitant way, that it wouldn't be so bad for him if I could jump into the pit with him. He moaned and mumbled to himself, and then he got up quietly and started to pace the floor. He said he could not withstand the voices any longer: "I had to obey them. I must be going crazy. I know I am, and I can't face the terrifying pit that I'm staring at." He said he was angry because I was leading him into the pit and that death was better. He wanted to take me along to punish me. There was no better place for me than inside his bowels, where he knew there was only pus and blood, or inside the pit. He felt that in a moment he would let his fists fly, and then he said he was going to ask for whiskey again to chase these thoughts away. "Everything is coming to a head, but I know that I can't vomit any more and this is a bad sign. If you can't get rid of these terrible things in you, they eat you all up and kill you from the inside."

The nurse told me the next morning that Tom had taken seven $2\frac{1}{2}$ ounces of whiskey and was almost completely drunk. He had gone on his own to the closed ward and had stayed there. I went to see him, but he turned his back and soon fell asleep. After he woke up I went to see him again. He announced that he was going to kill himself. He asked me to give him a medication myself. When I gave him a shot of demerol, he felt better. "Why didn't you do this before, Doc? I don't take demerol for pain but because it soothes these horrible feelings. I need something to lean on, but I'm worried. I'm too much for you. You look tired. Can you take it, Doc?" I reassured him that I could, but I did not sound very convincing—even to myself. Later on he became confused and begged me for something that would put him to sleep. However, he went to sleep soon afterward, without any medication.

CHAPTER X

DESPAIR AND CHAOS

FOLLOWING the episodes described in the previous chapter, which covered some three months, Tom's behavior changed. From now on he deteriorated precipitantly. Although he tried valiantly to fight back, he steadily lost ground, became more and more depressed, voiced suicidal inclinations, and stated that death was better than "the pit." When I asked him to describe this pit to me, he mumbled something about "a black nothing" that created a "feeling of doom" within him. The feeling of helplessness he seemed able to describe more easily. He said it was as if he were totally defenseless—that once he was in the pit there would be no way for him to get out and he would be at the mercy of "horrible things."

One day it was noted that he was shaking badly and was unable to answer questions. Yet, later that day, he explained the attack by saying that he had been seized with a terror that had "paralyzed his will" and that he was going to kill himself just to avoid facing this "black horror."

On another occasion he was found to be in a semi-stuporous state and could not be aroused. When, hours later, the nurse told me he was awake, I went at once to see him. He was barely able to recognize me. He mumbled something about having swallowed a female who was like a ball of fire inside him. He asked for whiskey to drown the fire that was eating him up. He made abortive efforts to vomit. He appeared completely confused. I tried to talk to him, but apparently he did not hear me. For the next two days, despite the fact that he had only six 50 mg. doses of demerol and very little alcohol, and retorted to what seemed to be accusatory voices, he managed to escape from his room and attempted to choke a woman patient who was sitting in her room; then, suddenly realizing what he was doing, he screamed in horror and returned quietly to his own room. Later on that day he attempted to make a rope out of his bed sheets in order to hang himself. Although he was under constant supervision, he managed once to run to the bathroom and tried to drown himself by putting his head into the toilet bowl.

In view of all this, plus his constant efforts to vomit which resulted in dehydration, we decided to give the patient only milk. He took a few sips, but again tried to vomit. Unaware of his surroundings, he paced the floor of his room, mumbling that he did not want to jump into the pit and that it was better to die. He begged one of the nurses, as if it were within her power to protect him, never to let him go into the pit because he feared he would not get out again. Despite his being sedated, he was extremely tense and restless. At times he ran round and round his room; then he would stop and stare at the floor, saying, "The black rocks! It is black in there—it is chaos in there—it is nothing." He kept repeating the words "chaos," "black," "nothing," as if this were the only way to describe the threat that caused his terror. His constant attempts to vomit out what he thought were the people he had swallowed reduced his strength. He would collapse in his bed and then suddenly get up and run to the nurses, asking for matches to light up "the fumes" that were coming out of his mouth. He was incontinent of urine and on one occasion was found smearing feces about his room, giving the appearance of a chronically hospitalized psychotic patient. Then he would ask for a drink of water to quench the fires inside him.

Tom remained in this confused and agitated state for three days. On the fourth day he appeared to be a little better. He was able to eat solid food for the first time in four days. With tears in his eyes, he came to me to tell me that it was his aunt whom he had swallowed.

TOM: She is right inside me and burning me up. I try to throw her up but I can't do it and I get mad. Then suddenly I saw her. There she was—my aunt, sitting quietly on the chair with her back turned to me. I felt suddenly strong. I knew I could grab her by the throat and squeeze her to death. I went slowly behind her. She didn't move. I put my hands on her neck. She laughed and said, "What are you doing, Tom? Stop kidding." I saw red. Her voice hadn't changed—always telling me off, giving me orders. I squeezed her neck, but she started to scream. The nurse and the orderly were at once upon me pulling my arms. I had to give up. Then she turned and looked at me. It was Mrs. G. I couldn't believe it! Good old Mrs. G., my friend. Oh Doc, what horrors! What's happening to me? Where am I going?
DOCTOR: Come on, Tom, give me your hand. Let's go into your room. [Tom followed me quietly. When we were both inside his room, I closed the door.] Tom, you cannot get out of this room from now on.

He started to cry. I went out and got a glass of milk and held it close to his mouth. He grabbed it and swallowed its contents in a gulp. He sighed, saying, "It soothes me for a while. It makes me feel human again." But that same afternoon he again became confused and untidy, and attempted to commit suicide by banging his head against a wall. He spent most of that night vomiting; finally, from sheer exhaustion, he went quietly to sleep.

At this point there was one encouraging feature—Tom's

insistent demands for medications decreased considerably. He did ask for demerol injections, but he would almost immediately forget that he had requested them. During this period I was able to cut down his demerol from 50 mg. to 5 mg., which meant an average of only seven to ten injections daily, in contrast with the huge amounts he had been receiving before. His demands for whiskey varied. Sometimes he would have none at all, and on other occasions he would drink heavily. During this time, fortunately, the infection in his abdomen seemed to be somewhat better, and the discharge from the anal area had subsided.

Despite his confusion, Tom's relationship with me remained on a friendly basis most of the time. He recognized me, appeared pleased to see me, and continued to express concern about my health. But his lucid intervals became less frequent and his hallucinatory periods more and more prolonged. On one of his better days he again asked for lobster, but when the nurse offered him some he refused it, saying that only milk would help him now. He also said he did not want any more demerol or whiskey. When I told him that I had taken him off barbiturates and had cut down his demerol to 5 mg. per injection because I thought he did not need it any more, he appeared pleased, but immediately asked whether I approved of his drinking. I answered that as far as I was concerned he could eat all he wanted, but that I hoped he would drink milk rather than whiskey. He smiled and made a motion as if waving good-bye. Later that same day, I was told that he wanted to talk to me. I found him crouched in bed. He did not answer when I spoke to him and soon started to moan. It was a moan that grew more and more high-pitched, until it sounded like an infant crying. I remained with him for a long time, but I was unable to get any other response from him, only this whining cry.

The next day Tom was a little more responsive. He told

me he could not remember what had happened to him during the past few days. He said he was horrified when he was told that he had attempted to strangle one of the patients. He remembered vaguely seeing the face of a woman and hearing "an echo from the past." At that moment his face became flushed. He looked furious and said, "I got a fit in my body. I grabbed her. I knew I hated her and I had to do it because she was responsible for my being in the pit. She was my aunt." I reminded him that we had talked about it before, but he had forgotten it completely. Later on that same day, he complained of hearing a very loud noise that was becoming so strong he could not stand it and was going to kill himself to avoid hearing it. He complained of blind spots in front of his eyes and the inability to focus on anything: "I know I am going blind, but blindness is better than the pit." He asked for a drink of whiskey in order to forget.

For the next two days Tom continued to drink very heavily. He took a total of between 15 and 20 ounces of whiskey per day and maintained a state of perpetual intoxication. He exposed himself several times, made threatening remarks to the nurses—"All women are to blame for my being in this pit"—and then became confused again. I went to see him and reminded him that he was confined to his room while he was drinking; but he looked blankly at me, not seeming to understand what I was saying.

I was called at one o'clock the next morning by the night nurse, who said that Tom wanted to see me. I went to him at once and spent the rest of that night and the whole of the next day with him. He was awake all this time and talked constantly. He said he was going to sleep in a pit to which there was no end. "There is no end to it and I'm ready to get in it," he said. "It is filled with dark rocks and there is a crack in the middle that signifies death." He avoided lying in his bed because he said it was his deathbed. "It is my aunt who is lying dead on my mattress," he said. He dragged the mattress off his bed and threw it onto the floor. My supervisor and I were disturbed by these demonstrations of the patient's withdrawal, and we decided that I should begin to feed him myself in an effort to help him through his ordeal. During all this time I continued to offer him milk. At first he refused it and turned his back on me, but after a while he appeared to understand and accepted some of it. He said he was going in and out of the pit, and was getting accustomed to it, and that it did not seem so frightening any more. He said there were terrifying things in there, but that death was a way he had discovered to avoid the pit.

Tom talked very little during the rest of this particular period, but he remained completely dependent upon me and seemed to be very grateful for my care. He continued to make the moaning sounds, but whenever I approached him he would smile. He held my hand for a long time one day and finally said he would do anything for me—even get inside the pit, with its music and its rocks—because he knew I was going to give him a hand and try to help him get out.

After this long interlude of two weeks, Tom appeared to be somewhat better. One morning Mrs. N., the discharged patient to whom he had been so attached, came to visit him. He seemed relaxed and contented while she was with him, but after her departure he again showed signs of confusion and complained that he had been abandoned. It was not long before he was back in his old depressed state, "full of destruction" and announcing that he was ready to die because no one cared for him and he was surrounded by feelings of loneliness and death. When I went to see him, he said, "I am going to dive into a sea of bubbles. This is the best way out." When I asked where this sea of bubbles was, he answered that it was inside the pit. He again said he was terrified to go into the pit because he knew he would never get out again, and he repeated that it was preferable to die—to kill himself in order to avoid it. I made the decision to stay with Tom as much as I could from then on, and I told him I was going to feed him his milk myself. Every time I went to see him, I offered him milk in a baby bottle. The first time I did this he produced a dollar bill and gave it to me, saying this was a token of his deep appreciation because it was his only possession in the world. I told him I realized this and added that I was sure we would win together. After this, Tom fell asleep. He slept for twelve hours. I also slept the same length of time.

During the next few days Tom was in better spirits. The only food he took was milk, but he was able to sleep much of the time. He did not ask for whiskey, but continued to request demerol off and on. Actually, his decision to give up whiskey occurred under the following arrangement: I told the nurse to give him whiskey every time he asked for it, but to offer him a bottle of milk along with it. Every time he asked me for whiskey, I also offered him milk. Finally he smiled and said he understood what we were all trying to do for him. "Whiskey is death and milk is life," he said. As I mentioned before, I had cut down the demerol medication to 5 mg. per injection, but when Tom gave up the whiskey on his own I decided to increase his demerol to 50 mg. since he had again started to complain of pain. During the next eight days his demands for medication varied from a minimum of nine to a maximum of seventeen 50 mg. injections for every twenty-four-hour period.

This temporary improvement did not last as long as I had hoped it would. On one occasion Tom told me that he was killing himself. He said he could not tolerate the pit and that he could now see things clearly. When I asked him what he meant, he said he could see a casket very plainly and wondered why I could not see it. In addition, he said he could hear voices constantly and was unable to shut them off. "I am absolutely at the mercy of these voices and lights," he said. At this time I began to wonder whether, because of the visual hallucinations, delirium tremens might be developing, but I dismissed the possibility because there was no other clinical manifestation of that disorder.

During the next week Tom remained in a withdrawn and depressed state. One month had gone by since he had been put on the closed ward for the first time, and, generally speaking, he was unmistakably deteriorating mentally. He was angry at everyone and complained to me that I had taken away his whiskey. When I reminded him that "whiskey is death," he smiled. I also told him that I could not go along with him in his self-destructive wishes. He appeared to accept this and did not continue to ask for whiskey. However, he sank deeper and deeper into a dependent state. He also assumed the behavior of an infant. He wore his surgical bandages like diapers, and he lay all day in bed, staring into space. When milk was offered to him, he would respond with childish sounds that were meant to express gratitude. The nurses fed him milk from a bottle as they would have fed a baby.

Soon, however, serious medical complications arose—severe inguinal lymphangitis with a resulting massive edema of the lower extremities and penis. It appeared that again his infection had flared up and was rapidly getting out of control. Cultures taken revealed growth of B Proteus, Staphylococcus aureus, and Beta hemolytic streptococcus; all three were resistant to penicillin and streptomycin, but showed growth inhibition by the use of chloromycetin. The medical service was called into consultation; they suspected a pelvic thrombophlebitis. The surgical service could offer no specific help.

Tom did not seem to pay much attention to these new complications. On the contrary, there was a hypomanic element in his mood. He quickly emerged from his withdrawn state and talked in grandiose terms about how he was going to overcome his new difficulties and was going to drive the devil out and completely recover. He professed great confidence in himself, and in his eyes I was the best doctor he had ever had because I did what he wanted. He said he did not worry because he was convinced that his troubles were already over. He slept a great deal—ten, twelve, fourteen hours out of twenty-four. When he was awake he was in good spirits. He was even allowed to go visiting in the open ward.

We decided to follow the advice of the medical service and start the patient on chloromycetin, which we hoped would eliminate his infections and decrease the edema. When I told Tom about the new drug, he did not appear to be disturbed, but later on that day I noticed a definite change in his demeanor. He suddenly became very depressed and again started to moan and to demand medication. He complained of an inability to swallow. He said that the same thing had happened to his father and that this symptom had caused his father's death. He wondered how frightened his father had felt when he was spitting blood and could not swallow. His father must have been scared of "his pit," he said, and this was the reason why his father's coffin was still inside the pit: "My father died and his torture was over, but I can't die and I have to face the torture of the pit." His voice sounded hollow and flat. He had the fantasy of plunging a knife into his aunt because her food was poison. His demand for medication increased. He was profoundly depressed, but his visual and auditory hallucinations had disappeared. Despite marked improvement in his physical condition due to the chloromycetin therapy, his depression deepened. More and more he lay in bed in a semistuporous state. Making contact with him became practically impossible. He simply moaned, stared at the ceiling, and mumbled occasionally.

I spent all my free time with him, but he made no effort to communicate with me. At times he lay utterly motionless in bed for hours. He was a living dead person. He had to be fed intravenously or by tube. The infection and the edema subsided rapidly, but he continued to be unresponsive. It was as if an enormous wall had descended between us. I visited him with my supervisor, and we repeatedly told him that we were alarmed because he was trying slowly to kill himself. He paid no attention to us. It seemed as if there was nothing else I could do to pull him out of this state, though I kept on urging him to try to help himself. Once he mumbled that he was "no good" and that his body was disintegrating. Another time he repeated the words "mother" and "no love." Tom remained in this profound stupor for four days. He seemed to have entered the pit.

Chloromycetin therapy, in the meantime, was producing a medical miracle by reducing the patient's infection and bringing the sepsis under control. In one week the edema subsided and finally disappeared. A minor flare-up of infection, because of Proteus' resistance to chloromycetin, was treated with streptomycin and cleared up rapidly. Yet Tom remained withdrawn, uncommunicative, and semistuporous.

Then—one day, two weeks later, I found Tom awake and responsive. He sat up in bed and said, "It's over, Doc. I defeated the pit. It must be a miracle, but a new life is going to start now!" I was amazed by the sudden and radical change, but it seemed to be genuine. Tom appeared, somehow, to have emerged from the pit.

There was a great deal of fluctuation in Tom's condition between the time of his dramatic announcement that he had emerged from his psychological pit and the improvement in his infection and the disappearance of the edema. From now on, it was possible to approach him. He again became talkative and it was easy to communicate with him. During our visits together I tried to summarize for him what had happened during the period of his prolonged silence and how we had been frustrated by his withdrawal. I did not expect, of course, to have an intellectual discussion with him, but I hoped that during this lucid period he would at least try to tell me what had happened to him during the four days in the pit. I urged him to describe what he remembered.

Tom tried to answer my questions by saying that he had been in "the black pit." I told him that he had mentioned this black pit several times, but that it was impossible for me to know exactly what he meant. He had experienced a tremendous fear before entering the pit: "Fear is not the word for it," he said. "It was more than that. It was the end." He said he had felt sure that, despite my efforts to help him by giving him whatever medication and whiskey and food he wanted, all was lost. He had felt that he was being swallowed by quicksand and that he was going into a place where there was absolutely nothing. "Everything was black," he said. "This is why I called it a pit. It was like a void." He added that what was even worse for him was the fact that it was a torture, a "living hell." Death would have been a way out of it all. He said that he had been overcome by a murderous rage—a rage against the people who were responsible for his having to face such a frightening ordeal. The people who came to his mind at the time were all women—Mrs. N., his first girlfriend, his old woman friend, and finally his aunt. He said that at times he had doubted that I was on his side, and then he would realize that, despite my assurances, there was little I could do to help him. At times he had felt paralyzed with fear and then, in a desperate effort, he would try to fight back, but soon everything would become confused. He remembered the day he attacked the woman patient on the closed ward. He said he thought he was strangling his mother, who had brought him into a "world of helplessness." Killing the people who were responsible for his condition was a last resort. It was the only way to express his anger, to do something actively in his own behalf.

He tried to describe to me what this "fearful pit" was all about, and again he used the word "nothing." "It was a part of me, yet it wasn't. There was complete paralysis there. I was at the mercy of horrifying black shadows moving all around me, and I couldn't stir." This prospect was terrifying, and his fury toward the people who had abandoned him became overwhelming. He said that, when he was unable to make himself try to kill them, the thought of killing himself instead had suddenly appealed to him. Death was the easier solution, when compared with the agony of facing such horror. It was then that he had tried to put his head into the toilet bowl in an attempt to drown himself. He also described the voices that had constantly told him terrible stories about the pit and urged him to kill others and himself as well. "There is no hope in the pit for you, Tom. Kill, kill, kill! Do away with yourself. It's better to die than to face the pit—the black rocks, the fires, the horrors—when you are completely helpless and at the mercy of it all." He said he had been aware that I was around somewhere, trying to help him out of his predicament, but he felt that I, too, was a helpless person and was at the mercy of these same overwhelmingly powerful "things," that I was also going to be destroyed by the very things that threatened him. But on other occasions, he said, he had viewed me as attempting to stem this tide. I would appear strong, and his hopes would be revived—but not for long, because he would soon be filled again with the paralyzing fears.

Tom remembered that his efforts to combat the fear lasted for a long time. But one morning he suddenly felt that he was inside the pit. He could not explain how this happened. Suddenly the voices had stopped, and he saw that he was in the bottom of the black pit, with rocks all around him. Then there was a terrific noise, and at the end of a tortuous path there was his coffin. He said that this must have meant his death, but he was unable to move toward the coffin because death would deliver him from the living hell. From then on, he had lost track of time and of all that was happening. (This was the four days when he was in what looked like a profound stuporous state somewhat resembling a combination of retarded depression and catatonia.) He remembered awakening from this slumber on one occasion and realizing that his body had become "all puffed up and was falling to pieces"—it was the price he was paying for being in the pit. (This was how he perceived the period when he had developed massive edema in his extremities.) He could not account for the rest of the time. He said he could not think or act. "I was at the mercy of everything—noises, lights, pain—and I was unable to move. It was as if I was dead, yet alive, and not knowing what was happening to me. Finally, one day I woke up. It was like getting out of a tunnel and facing the sun for the first time." Then he noticed that he could move and that he could see color once more. The noises subsided, and the first words he remembered hearing clearly and understanding were mine: "Tom, we have won."

Now he felt alive again. There was hope. Everything started to come back to him. He could remember the hospital, the ward, the patients—yet it was all different. He had come back from a place that was impossible to describe. It was as if he had half-died and then returned to life. He felt that now he could think of the future. Things had changed, and he was going to try to get well and to go on living a new life.

After Tom stopped talking, I felt that he had just tried to describe something that was very unusual. His experience seemed to be unique. He could find no words to describe what had really happened to him, and I was amazed by this extraordinary story.

A few days later he gave me a three-page written report. He said that now he could remember a great deal about his special treatment and wanted me to know what he thought about it. Here are some excerpts from this report:

"I remember having a feeling inside me that told me, 'Your days are numbered.' At such times I felt a cold chill. Everyone I knew that had this operation is dead. I feel panicky. I rush to my doctor. The only way to fight such thoughts is by medication, by pain, yet my pain is not any worse. I get satisfied for a while from demerol, but I want whiskey instead. I get all the whiskey I want and then I want more. This is great! My doctor gives me the things I need. He is a fool, but maybe he has something up his sleeve. I am smart, too. I mix well with the other patients. I try to help everybody. I need Mrs. N.—this wonderful woman—to help me out. She has a magnetic personality. I am going to help her. I can do it. I can be a psychiatrist and more than that. She needs a good doctor. Her name has a sweet taste. I love her. I would love to kiss her lips and her breasts. My whole being cries for whiskey. Dr. S. knows how I feel. He is waiting and I must tell him about how I feel—yet I do not think I can do that. God! I want more whiskey. So I go to my doctor and tell him how wicked it is. Yet the thought that I have is that it is happening to me. What is he doing to me? I can have all I want now! He takes away my suffering, yet I want to punish him. I'll stop before I get too far—like hell. I have 16 nembutal capsules. I'll wait until I have more. I want to be sure I'll kill myself. I'll miss him. He gave me a good deal. Why do I think such things? I've got to play ball. He trusts me. I have got to give him back all this stuff. What the hell kind of a guy am I anyway? Here, Doc, take these nembutals.

"I'm sitting in a bathtub. I look at the pus running out of my body. My body is on fire. My backside is running and my penis and my testes are all infected. I am going to die. Nobody gives a good Goddam. The hell with them. I'll tell my doc to go to hell. He said he can do things to me. Let him try. I'm too smart for him. He said that if he does things they are for my own good. He is going to turn the heat on. Whatever you do to me, I'll take it. You can kill me if you want to. I can take it. Open the window, tell me to jump, and I'll go through. Try me. I can always win. He says, 'If you feel unsafe you can go to the closed ward. Just walk down and tell the nurses.' 'O.K.,' I say, 'but I'll kill you.' Then it is whiskey I want—whiskey. Help me drown the fire. My whole body is on fire. Fire. What an idea. I'll drink a whole glass of acetone. Light myself up. Rupture my lungs. Burn up like the fireworks on the 4th of July. No one can stop me. Power. I've got the power of death. It is mine. Mine, all alone. See, the doctor is helpless. Jesus, I'm strong. I'll pour out the acetone, open up the box of matches, and lay one on top of the box. I'll light it, hold it while I drink. Dr. S.'s voice comes back to me. 'You promised. How could you want to kill yourself?' I can't stand it any longer. The doctor comes to see me. 'Go on now, Tom, let me take you back to the closed ward.' Then I forget. Time goes by—the bathtub, the bubbles, soft bubbles, I want to breathe bubbles and go to sleep. I want to die. The doctor comes to me. His voice is screaming in my ear, 'Do you hear me? Wake up, drink a glass of water. Vomit, rinse your mouth, drink a glass of milk.' And then the pit. Pit, pain, fire, sickness, darkness, vacuum, sharp rocks, desolation. The doctor gives me a glass of milk. I realize that, with the exception of milk, I don't know what this is all about. I want to talk to my doctor and I want to drink something. Two glasses on the table. One is whiskey and one is milk. Which one to choose? Which one to take? Whiskey is poison and it means sickness, hatred and death. Milk is food, good food, and it means health, love and kindness. 'Drink something, Tom.' I hear his voice. 'Take your choice.' Something big here, I think. A hand reaches out. Milk. He wants me to drink milk. My hand picks the glass of milk. I drink slowly at first, and then like a child. It feels so good. The taste, it is an old taste. A taste I know. I hear the doctor's voice. 'We have won.' "

This mixed-up account was all that Tom could remember of the last two months in anaclitic treatment. When I asked him about his fear, he did not remember; nor did he recall his fury at women and his attempt to kill the woman patient. He viewed the treatment as a miracle that in some way I had performed by giving him milk. I thought that repression had set in, performing its merciful and therapeutic task by giving rise to amnesia. His elated mood quickly subsided, but in general he remained in good spirits.

I decided now that it was time to start imposing restrictions on the patient. I thought that Tom must have had a therapeutic experience because he felt better, and so it was appropriate for him to start learning the limits of everyday life. In a sense, what I was hoping to do was to re-educate him and help him to readjust to reality. I also believed that, since he had viewed me as someone who had stood by him throughout his ordeal, he would at least be convinced that he had not been abandoned by the person on whom he had depended so completely. I hoped that this experience could counterbalance some of his previous losses. There was also the slight possibility that he could learn once again to relate to people, without expecting an inevitable tragedy to result from the loss of a person he might attach himself to.

One week after his dramatic description of the pit, I asked Tom to come to my office for an interview. I told him then that we thought he should be ready to be discharged from the hospital in two months. I said that I was going to take back, from then on, full control of his medication and that there would be no more whiskey. He seemed to be startled at first, but then he smiled and said he was ready for anything. He was happy to live again: "Maybe I enjoyed the horrors somehow. You see, Doc, either way I win."

From now on his mood was an elated one. He was feeling fine—"better than at any other time in my life," he said. I was viewed as the "superhuman doctor who had performed a miracle that was unique in the history of medicine." I kept emphasizing that there had been no miracle, that he had faced his difficulties on his own, with my help. He said that the deadline given for his discharge from the hospital was a good idea. He was ready himself to make the supreme effort toward achieving "total success," and he felt convinced that, with my help, he would be cured. So in this way my rapport with the patient, which had been lost for such a long time, was rapidly re-established, and I was pleased to see Tom facing the future with so much confidence.

Tom was still receiving some demerol, but I was able to eliminate all medication in less than three weeks. He described this time as his "test period." Occasionally he was resentful and attempted to talk me into giving him demerol. He would ask for whiskey or for a special food from the new nurse on the ward. My answer to this was that he had to face this period of growing up and that, realistically, life required strict limitations on things like medication, alcohol, and privileges. One day Tom asked to see me. This was the last time that he was allowed to see me at his own request, because I had decided to give him only one regular interview daily. He said that all of a sudden he knew what had happened. He was reborn and he realized that it took time for a newborn baby to learn how to walk and talk, but that finally he would grow up into a big strong man who could stand on his own two feet. He understood why I was setting up all these limitations: "This is what a father does with his children." Again, on one occasion, he tried to get morphine from a new doctor who had just arrived from France, but Dr. C. knew all about the patient's situation and morphine was not given to him. The next day Tom mentioned during his interview with me that he was sure Dr. C. had been "briefed." Although he had thought of his father as never denying him anything, he realized now that he must learn that his new father had to deny him everything.

CHAPTER XI

REHABILITATION

BY THE END of about a month's time after the restrictions had been imposed, Tom's infection had cleared up completely. Chloromycetin, streptomycin, and penicillin all did their good work. So, at this point, I started to make arrangements for his discharge from the hospital. I asked him if he had any plans for the future, such as a job and a place to stay, and suggested that he talk about this with a social worker. After the first interview with the social worker, Tom became disturbed. He cried and told me he had the feeling that we wanted to get rid of him. He talked about the possibility of going to his brother's house and said he realized that he had problems in his marriage situation that had not in any way been changed. Thus he seemed to be more realistic in outlook.

For the next few days he appeared somewhat depressed. He complained that his infection was bothering him again, and that he was finding it difficult to keep up with the rigid demands we were placing on him. "It is hard to keep up with progress," he added. He again doubted his ability to overcome his infection. I told him that the infection had cleared up and that I thought he was asking for medication in a roundabout way. He admitted that this was so and asked for some "soothing demerol." The next day, for the first time, he told me that he had felt a great deal of resentment for me, but that he understood my position. He thought I was not as interested in him as I had been in the past: "Here is the evidence, Doc. You always used to carefully investigate my infected sores when I showed you the discharges, and you always gave me a complete physical examination. You haven't done this recently." I gave him my reasons for not doing this and again reminded him that his infection had cleared up. I also told him that, though I was still interested in him, the past had been the past and that now I had to convince him that I was on his side in trying to help him become more independent and to stand on his own feet. I reassured him that his infection was foremost in my mind and added that I was of greater help to him by giving him more freedom; I hoped he would start to make up his own mind and depend on me less. Finally I said, "The treatment was a successful experience—not only for you, Tom, but for me too." With that, he seemed to be satisfied.

As time went by, Tom became more self-confident. Working long hours in occupational therapy, he invented a more efficient ileostomy bag. I decided to cut down his privileges concerning special foods—the last such privileges he had. Tom, realizing that the period of free indulgence was drawing to a close, had again increased his demands and was eating excessive amounts of ice cream and other kinds of extra treats. He seemed resigned to my statement about the food restriction, though he made a last-minute attempt to persuade me to reconsider; finally he accepted my decision. I understood his wish to get back his old privileges, but I cautioned him about trying to return to a passive-dependent position because it would no longer be beneficial to him. I explained that the anaclitic treatment, with all the privileges, had been of great help to us once; but now he should be ready to accept responsibility because at the present time he had grown up enough to take matters into his own hands—an achievement we could not have believed possible three or four months earlier.

The next day Tom admitted that he had been testing me out and that he was quite satisfied with the hospital diet. He said he realized that every special privilege had to be stopped because it was incompatible with his progress. He also admitted that he had gorged himself with all those good foods. Although he was a little annoyed, he started to make plans for his discharge from the hospital. On one occasion he told me that he realized he was walking a very narrow path, but had confidence that this was the only way to get well.

During the next month I left for a two-week vacation. Tom was very apprehensive at first, since it was his first separation from me in eight months. We had talked about it for some time and had decided it was a good test of his progress. I said I was confident that he would be able to carry on very well without me. We made a specific appointment time for the exact day of my return. He was friendly and cooperative, made no demands for medication, and talked about his plans for the future. He planned to go and live for a while with a friend, who had once offered him a room. After he got a job, he would decide what to do next. This was peculiar because he had had a fight with this friend, and Tom claimed that he disliked the man very much and wanted to kill him when he was disturbed. When I asked him about it, he said that, although he had never felt very close to him, he could see no reason for turning down the friend's invitation. He had forgotten all about his rage at him. He showed me an ileostomy bag that he had finished at occupational therapy and gave it to me as a gift. It was an ingenious device. His spirits were good all that day.

During my vacation Tom was seen frequently by another doctor who had followed the treatment progress and was acquainted with the problems. At times Tom seemed upset and on occasion demanded medication. Once or twice he appeared to be depressed, but the situation was handled very well by the doctor.

When I returned, I found Tom in good spirits. He spoke at length about his experiences during my absence. He was angry, he said, because I had left no medication for him. When I reminded him that we had decided to cut it down and that he had agreed three weeks before, he smiled and said he was testing me. Actually, he seemed happy. He said he had missed his interviews with me, and at times thought I was not coming back; but he had soon dismissed such thoughts. He had managed to be pleasant to the nurses and the other patients on the ward. He said, with a smile, that he had continued to make plans for the future. At the end of the interview, he asked me if I would trust him to go across the street to buy some tobacco. I gave him permission to go, which made him very happy. It was the first time he had gone out of the hospital in a period of seven months. He dressed himself up, and all the nurses admired him and made quite an occasion out of it. He thanked me, saying that he was impressed by my trust in him. He was out for an hour.

From now on, Tom was given ground privileges, which he used very wisely. The social worker noticed a great change in him. She thought at first that he had only been making plans, but that now he had really decided to get involved in finding a job. We decided that, although he was still somewhat tense, he was better than he had ever been in the past year. He remained cheerful for the next three weeks, and the date for his discharge was set.

During his last week in the hospital, Tom showed some animosity toward the hospital and toward the social worker for making plans for his discharge. He talked to me about it in an indirect way. I told him that this animosity was primarily directed at me and that I understood how he felt.

I said it was natural to be angry after such a long stay in the hospital, and I encouraged him to speak freely with me about his feelings. I added that I knew he was ready to face life on his own, because I had confidence in him and knew he would succeed. We shook hands.

Before his discharge, Tom was presented to the psychiatry staff conference of the Massachusetts General Hospital and was interviewed by the chief of service. He was in a jubilant mood and talked at great length about his treatment. He referred to it several times as a "miracle" and expressed his gratitude for having been helped to "begin a new life." When he was asked about the future, he described his plans in great detail. After he left the room, his case was discussed by several members of our department, and the consensus of opinion was that he had been helped.

The patient had been hospitalized in the psychiatry department for a little more than a year. He was discharged as planned, and I saw him in the psychiatry clinic off and on for a period of six months. His elated mood continued, and he talked much about the miracles that had been performed and referred to his therapist as a "superhuman being" who had given him a new life. In his visits to the clinic, he would spend most of the time talking about the self-confidence he had acquired, although he admitted there would be difficulties that he would have to encounter and conquer. He often spoke about looking for a job. He said he felt that he did not need any further psychotherapy. Most of it had already been done, he thought, but he wanted to come to see me occasionally just to say hello. Six months later he appeared to be in good spirits.

During the next nine years I saw Tom six times. As was expected, he had been obliged to face enormous problems in his life. His relationship with his wife and his family improved somewhat, but the problems with his ileostomy and difficulties he encountered in getting a job were complex. Immediate demands were placed on him for the support of his family. Although physically and mentally he was able to work, he felt discouraged. I saw him on two occasions in 1958. He was in good spirits, but he talked about the difficulties associated with the realities of the everyday life he was caught up in. He seemed, as always, to be enthusiastic about his experiences in the hospital and expressed a great deal of gratitude for me. He said he would have been dead if it had not been for the treatment he had received, that he had had seven years of living he had not counted upon, and that this had been the most worthwhile period in his life. Around the spring of 1959, I heard that he was medically ill and had been hospitalized on two occasions.

I saw Tom in September 1960 and noticed a marked change in his appearance. He was a discouraged man. He was living with his wife and children but, because of repeated infection owing to poor hygiene of his ileostomy, he had been unable to work. He remembered the anaclitic relationship as "a miracle" that gave him "many good years of life." When I pointed out that it had been no miracle but an attempt to help him out of a difficult position, he simply smiled. I asked him for permission to write about his anaclitic treatment. He smiled, "Doc, you must write your side of it because it is the scientific side, and it must be known, but please make it sound human. Don't put in big words that are hard to understand. Make it alive. Try to show to people what it's like to be in hell and how there is a way of getting out, and most important of all please write about the two of us." I promised to try. A few days later I received his letter giving me full authorization to go ahead with my description of our joint experience.

I saw him again in May 1961. Now in his late forties, he looked well and seemed to be in good spirits. We had coffee together—talking and reminiscing for over an hour. Tom said that he had come to the hospital to visit an old friend who had been admitted the previous night. He said that he had tried to reassure his friend by giving him a long lecture about the history of the hospital. He added, "I told him that this was the place where miracles happened. It was here that ether was first used as an anesthetic; it was here that they learned to treat burns." Then smiling at me, he added, "It was here that they brought Tom back from the dead." Two days later I learned that Tom had died suddenly and painlessly in his sleep, of a coronary occlusion.

Toward the end of the unique, bizarre, and often frustrating experience, I had begun to realize that I felt a very special affection for Tom. I had learned to admire his wit, his struggles, and his courage. I miss him.

DISCUSSION

ONE OF the most important aspects of this case was the relationship between the patient's physical and psychological symptoms. The psychological symptoms seemed to improve when his physical condition deteriorated and to deteriorate when his physical condition improved. (This has been observed in other patients with psychosomatic diseases, but exactly why it occurs is still unknown.) Tom's early depression, followed by auditory hallucinations, and the increased alcohol intake, which seemed to be an attempt to react to these two symptoms, developed for the first time after he had recovered from his first surgical operation and had become physically well. These psychiatric symptoms interfered quickly with his general functioning, and hospitalization in the psychiatry service became imperative. In this proper setting and with the help of his second psychiatrist, Tom's mental state quickly improved. He was moved from the closed to the open ward, where he mingled amicably with the other patients; but soon there developed ulcerations in the blind pouch of the sigmoid and rectum that had been left behind following his operation. After the second operation he did fairly well from the physical point of view; but then he started to deteriorate psychiatrically and became so addicted to demerol that it was again necessary to transfer him to the psychiatry ward.

One of the difficulties throughout this patient's hospitalization was the problem of medication. It was because of his addiction to demerol, more than anything else, that the decision to prescribe narcotics freely was the most difficult one for me to make. To surrender such a privilege to a patient seemed like folly at the time; but Tom maintained his previous level of dosage for a while and his demands for medication did not even increase. It was only later, when faced with the overwhelming fears about the pit, that his demands for demerol or alcohol increased again. Taking away the drug to which a patient is addicted may not always be a wise course of action. Tom's suspicions and anger were always associated with the fear that I would deprive him of his medication. He seemed to use the demerol more to calm himself down than to alleviate his pain, and he talked about demerol as "soothing" his desperate loneliness and hostility. At the time when his infections were completely out of control, when he developed edema of his lower extremities and penis, when his legs were three times their normal size, not once did he ask for demerol; and later on he was willing, at first cautiously and then rapidly, to give up all forms of medication.

The antagonism shown by several nurses, and even by some members of the medical staff, toward our allowing the patient to have all the narcotics he wanted was quite amazing. Even when it was obvious that Tom was asking for less medication than he had before the anaclitic therapy started, the head nurse continually attempted to avoid giving him what he requested. The patient's anger and frustration with such delaying tactics were certainly justified.

Although the punitive position taken by the head nurse may be attributed to her own rigid personality, it is in a way characteristic of the majority of people who deal with alcoholics or drug addicts. The results of the treatment of alcoholism and drug addiction are notoriously unsatisfactory. One wonders to what extent this comes from the emphasis on withdrawing the alcohol or the narcotics, rather than on finding a substitute for the patient's frustrated dependent needs. Are the constant repetitious demands of such patients exasperating to people around them? Or is it, as well, the necessity to conform to "principle and dogma," as the head nurse put it, that makes some people anxious when they are challenged? I suppose that this need to conform can provide so much comfort and security that it gives rise to suspicion of any new attitude, which is viewed as dangerous and is resented vigorously. Such conformity stifles originality.

As far as the anaclitic relationship was concerned, it produced a change that seems to have occurred almost from the very beginning. The patient's reactions turned from those of suspicion and anger for his therapist to cautious cooperation and questioning trust. But was this apparent change evidence of an improved relationship? This is debatable. The original anger for me was associated with the departure of his previous therapist. After the establishment of a relationship with me, he seemed to express antagonism when he talked about liking the women patients on the ward and of being afraid that I would get angry at him for this and retaliate. He pretended that this was a friendly competition, but there was nothing friendly about it since he was unable to have good feelings for anyone for a long period of time. It was when he had regressed further, then, that this stage was followed by a passive-dependent period with an emergence of strong ambivalent feelings.

Tom seemed to feel that the only way in which he could deal with his antagonistic feelings for me was by surrendering passively and assuming a feminine role. What I am referring to here is his preoccupation with fantasies of being a woman: his behavior when, for example, he showed me his chest and claimed that he had "a big breast" which he expected should be cut off; or when he pointed to his abdo-

men and referred to it as "a big pregnant belly" and had the
fantasy that he could have been married to me. Finally, there
was the dramatic exhibition of the bloody towel and his associations to menstruation, which preceded the increase of
his alcohol intake. As fantasies of this nature became more
frequent, he started to become more and more anxious.
Unable to deal with this anxiety, he retreated further, thus
becoming helpless and needing to be even more dependent
than before. It was at this point that he became sensitive to
separations and began to talk about the people who had
abandoned him. Fear and anger, from then on, were the
predominant emotions. The more he talked about these feelings, the more disturbed he became, until he needed to rely
almost entirely upon his therapist. Therefore, it seems that
hostile dependence was the main aspect of the anaclitic relationship up to the time of Tom's emergence from the pit.
Afterward it was an exaggerated magical idolization.

Tom liked to challenge the rules and to fight the restrictions placed on him. It is true that he had encountered people
in the past who were willing to understand and to help
him, but he realized that they also were social outcasts who
were fighting a losing battle. He had put up a good fight
against society, and in this struggle he had had some temporary successes, such as the time when he held his own in
the argument with the priest, or when he was unwilling to
sign his name authorizing the adoption of his children; but
in the end, unwilling to compromise, he had been defeated.
His condition deteriorated rapidly, and from then on he
started to fall apart both physically and mentally.

He was particularly vulnerable to loss because his father
and grandmother died relatively soon after he had established some kind of relationship with them. The loss of his
uncle and two psychiatrists during his adult life repeated
this pattern. Finally, distrustful of human contacts, it was

almost easier for him to hate people than to be attached to them. Having established an anaclitic relationship, he was faced again with frustrating anger and overwhelming fear of loss. The more he became afraid, the more he needed his therapist; yet the irony of it was that, to get better, he had to face these emotions alone and had to have the courage to learn to live with them. Anaclitic support at this stage simply underlined to him his total helplessness. It was only a method for showing him a road to recovery, but it could not perform a miracle. The change had to come from him. This was the period that the patient described so dramatically and that turned out to be the most fascinating aspect of his therapy.

It seemed to him that he had to face the prospect of utter loneliness, with terrible fears of the unknown, and, at the same time, the frustrating rage of agonizing helplessness. This is what he described as the pit, and he made desperate efforts to evade it. Had he experienced such feelings some time long before? He tried to blame others, particularly people who had abandoned him—his family, his first girl-friend, and Mrs. N., the ward patient—for the predicament he was in. His fear fed his fury at these people until the idea of harming them appealed to him. In desperation he turned against his aunt, whom he blamed for all his troubles and whom he tried to attack in the person of the woman patient he assaulted when he was on the closed ward. But all this was of no avail. On other occasions his fury turned inward, and he tried to kill himself in order to get out of the trap he found himself in. As a third alternative, he attempted desperately to alter his environment, to distort it by denying it, just to escape the unbearable fright he was experiencing at the time. One could observe the psychotic delusions and hallucinations resulting from these abortive attempts to change reality. But nothing seemed to help. He somehow sensed that there was only one solution, and so he plunged finally into his pit. Confused, stuporous, uncommunicative, and totally alone, he erected a wall around him—he was stripped of all his defenses and at the mercy of his own most violent fury. In this profound state of retarded withdrawal, he found himself, or perhaps he recognized himself as he really was—a totally frightened being. But the psychotic symptoms, his homicidal and suicidal ideas, ceased. He needed no more narcotics, no more alcohol.

It is not clear how much Tom was aware of what was happening around him throughout this time. He did seem to notice that I was close to him, trying very hard to get in touch with him, and that he was not being left entirely alone. This was probably reassuring, but whether it helped him is questionable. His concurrent physical improvement may have triggered his ascent from the pit.

One must also consider all of this from another point of view. The anaclitic relationship implied an unrealistic satisfaction of all the patient's needs. Following the removal of his colon, this basically insecure and angry patient was able to deal with his rage by blaming the outside world and by making others his persecutors; after this he had to defend himself by fantasies, delusions, and thoughts of protecting himself by attacking others, as in the episode in the shipyards. His basic insecurity was thus relieved. In other situations he attached himself in a hostile, dependent manner to individuals who could support him by gratifying some of his needs, like his old woman friend and his psychiatrist. But any attempt on their part to frustrate him or to leave him immediately mobilized his wrath, which was expressed by a murderous rage toward them. Examples of this may be seen in his anger toward his first therapist, whom he wanted to attack after the psychiatrist had left him, despite a close four-year relationship; and the episode of smashing the lamp, thinking that the face of his second psychiatrist could be seen in it, despite his professed love for him at the time of their separation.

As mentioned before, Tom's relationship with me was at first characterized by hostility and suspicion, but when I offered to satisfy all his demands he was taken aback. He thought there must be a "catch" somewhere, but when he realized that I meant to offer him all the demerol he needed, a goal that he had never expected to achieve and that colored favorably our initial relationship, he switched his tactics and started to make unrealistic demands for expensive imported foods. Not expecting that these would be granted, he could be justified in blaming me, as he blamed the nurses, for not really wanting to help him. He was again taken aback, however, when he got what he asked for; again he became frustrated. Then he switched to alcohol, making that dramatic request at a most inopportune moment for me and involving me in its execution. He expected a rejection, in order to feel justified in projecting his anger and appearing as a helpless victim. But again this mechanism of projection was undercut, leaving him in a situation of demanding more and more of the impossible. When Tom finally demanded that I be with him all the time and give him constant support, thus using utter dependence as an ultimate weapon, my acceptance of this final challenge left him in agony—in a state of confusion resulting from his inability to project his anger—and looking furiously for a way out. In despair, as a final act of aggression, a gesture of total defiance, he withdrew himself to the horrors of his pit. Here he had to see himself as nothing more than a human being full of hate.

From this, one may view the anaclitic relationship as threatening to the patient. Our good will and our efforts to persuade him to trust us emotionally may have been effective in a completely different way from anything we were aware of at the time. Having succeeded in undercutting the patient's use of his predominant defense mechanism, we had forced him to face his full wrath and see himself as he really was—something he had never allowed himself to do before. In this way his anaclitic dependence was not the helpless dependence of an infant upon his mother, as one may have expected, since it has been thought to occur frequently in patients with ulcerative colitis. Instead it was a hostile dependence that offered the patient a way of expressing his rage, and in this sense it implied attempts at control and demonstrated a kind of strength, not weakness. Maybe this strength contributed to the patient's final victory over his fury and fear and led him to return to the reality of the outside world.

Looking at all of this from still a different point of view, it should be remembered that both Tom and I were helpless and hopeless. It is possible that this desperate state played an important role in motivating us to try something dramatically new, like the anaclitic therapy, and to work equally hard to make it succeed. Tom was a very sick patient who, physically and mentally, was going down hill, and it seemed that there was nothing we could do medically or psychologically to arrest the deterioration. Both the patient and the doctor were in despair, which is, according to some existentialists, the only true human condition. Perhaps, in this predicament, we could understand each other better than we could have otherwise. The conviction that any improvement was only temporary, that inevitably there would be an exacerbation of difficulties, that the problem we faced was insoluble, that, even if Tom could improve somewhat in the hospital, he would always have to return to exactly the same social situation and environment from which he had come and which would rapidly bring about another catastrophe—all this emphasized strongly that the

only thing that counted was the "here and now." Thus I
had to concentrate on the day-to-day routine rather than on
future plans. From Tom's statements, quoted here, it is clear
that he was aware of his own despair. But what is more
striking was his awareness of my desperate frustration. He
mentioned at times that he was worried about me and was
concerned about my health. Because we were confronting
one another fully aware that we were both in the same boat,
it is possible that we developed an ability to share each
other's misery. And from this emerged a better understanding of one another, which, in the form of the anaclitic relationship, helped us to take a constructive step in the right
direction.

Whatever the reason for his re-establishing of contact
with reality, Tom seemed to change. He appeared rejuve-
nated and talked about a new life. His conscious attempts
to delay "growing up" were few; most of the time he co-
operated fully and his rehabilitation proceeded rapidly. The
somewhat elated mood that prevailed during this time did
not interfere with our plans for his discharge. Yet there was
no evidence that Tom had changed in any basic way as far
as his relations to other people were concerned—that he was
willing to give more than he would receive. There was,
however, a definite change in his mood, in his feeling of
general well-being and self-esteem.

Is there a parallel between Tom's experiences and those
of psychotic, homicidal, and suicidal patients? In one study
at the Massachusetts General Hospital of patients who have
attempted suicide,[1] it was demonstrated that some of them
seemed to have tried to look back on their lives in a desperate
attempt to find something worthwhile and satisfactory; but,

[1] P. E. Sifneos, C. Gore, and A. C. Sifneos, "A Preliminary Psychiatric
Study of Attempted Suicide as Seen in a General Hospital," *American
Journal of Psychiatry*, 112:883–888 (May 1956).

at the moment before the suicidal attempt, everything looked overwhelmingly black and death appeared as the logical answer—the appropriate exit, the perfect way out. They did not seem preoccupied with what it would be like to be dead, but much more concerned with how to get rid of their miserable and painful lives. These patients viewed suicide as the one and only way to alleviate pain and to solve their emotional problems. When Tom talked about suicide, he also mentioned that his life was full of pain. Death appeared to him as a merciful solution. "Thank goodness there is death," he said.

Some patients who have attempted suicide used their suicidal attempt as a way to manipulate others in a desperate effort to go on living. It appeared impossible for them to brave the likelihood of life without their loved ones. Facing loneliness, along with hostility, they decided to solve their problem by killing themselves, or to use suicide as a powerful last-minute act in order to manipulate the environment and regain the lost person.[2] When some of these patients are interviewed the day after an effective manipulative suicidal attempt, one is surprised to find them almost jubilant. They seem to have discovered the power that suicide commands as a weapon of social maneuver and do not seem to be motivated to receive psychotherapy.[3]

Tom also on some occasions thought of suicide as a way to manipulate other people, including his therapist, in an effort to get from us what he wanted. But he was able to understand what he was doing, and this insight led to his

[2] P. E. Sifneos and W. F. McCourt, "A Study of the Mode and Motive of Some Patients Who Attempted Suicide," *Proceedings of the Third World Congress of Psychiatry* (Toronto: University of Toronto and McGill, 1962), pp. 1245–1250.

[3] P. E. Sifneos, "Manipulative Suicide, Preliminary Observations," in preparation.

returning to me the barbiturate pills that he had collected. However, one should not forget those who kill themselves because their honor is at stake, or those who are too confused or depressed to realize what they are doing. It is useful to classify patients into meaningful categories, but it should be remembered that every attempt at self-destruction or destruction of another human life is a complicated, idiosyncratic act which must always be understood on an individual basis. It should give us no consolation to know that a devout Catholic Italian father of six children, who threatened to take his own life and did succeed in killing himself, happened to have defied sociological theories about suicide.

Are all of these patients trying to avoid a regression, a pit of their own, in their final attempt to recapture their lost loved ones? Are some of the people who kill others, or attempt to, and end up in prison rather than in a hospital, facing their own pit? What happened while Tom was in the pit? The feelings that predominated before his withdrawal were utter loneliness, pure hate, and dread of the unknown. This was coupled with almost a motor paralysis. His behavior seemed to indicate from then on extreme sensitivity to sensory stimuli. Battered from within by a sensory bombardment of lights and noises, he was nevertheless unable to react against it.

Tom was unable to talk about the state he was in because he could not find the words to describe it adequately. He used terms such as "desolation," "vacuum," "pit," "black," "nothing," to communicate his helplessness in dealing with what he felt was an overwhelming assault upon him. Yet this assault originated within himself—he tried to blame the outside world, but could not do this for long. He put up a good fight and preferred death to the dreaded horrors, but in despair or in defiance he had the courage to plunge into his pit. In his own words: "When you hit the bottom, there is no other way you can go but back up again." Hope thus emerged from chaos.

Whatever it was, one may speculate that experiencing these powerful frustrations, with the resulting fury, dread, and hopelessness, ultimately contributed to the change in his behavior and mood. Would Tom from then on be less vulnerable to separations? Would he in some way be immunized against such exigencies? Was it a deprived beginning of life, with his genetic inheritance, his early conditioning to his environment, his illness, his traumatic separations, that made him more liable as an adult to develop psychosis, drug addiction, alcoholism, and wishes to kill others and himself? Is this what happens to others who develop such traits and, if so, why? Is a dread of the unknown the first and basic experience for them all, with the emotions of love and anger only secondary to it? Are these emotions attempts to find a way to overcome it? Do repeated frustrations of these feelings lead back to the facing of this horrible dread all over again? Is it loss of a loved one that threatens young children more than anything else? Are some adults who have been vulnerable, because of loss, likely to regress until they face the threat of utter helplessness and experience the agonies of the unknown? Was Tom one of these people? Or is it all aggression in the first place? It is hard to answer these questions from the material available, but one may speculate.

Dread of the unknown is an experience that one encounters in children and hears patients talk about very often, but it is hard to know what is meant exactly by such a term. In some patients, like Tom, life requires constant effort. It seems to be a continuous terror, which at times reaches enormous proportions, particularly when they have to face the unknown—their own pit. Death—or better, nonbeing—is viewed as supremely blissful and serene, a Nirvana-like state that goes on and on, uninterrupted and undisturbed. Tom sought death and was never afraid of it. When he was close to death, he showed remarkable courage. Since life itself became dread of the unknown, it was a perpetual misery; anything that remotely or temporarily alleviated the pain was viewed as a great happiness. Any kind of pleasure, then, is given a very high priority, and fear of its loss is vigorously reacted against. The emotion of love is quickly equated with pleasure; the emotion of anger is quickly aroused when pleasure is threatened. Thus, separations from loved ones are deeply painful experiences. As a young human being grows up, he must learn to deal with love, with fears of the loss of pleasures, and with the ensuing anger that one associates with each stage in his emotional development. It is possible, of course, to imagine that an infant who has inherited a tendency to hyperactivity, like the restless baby one commonly sees in the nursery of a lying-in hospital, will be easily frustrated during the first few weeks of his life. If his family environment exposes such an infant to only a few frustrations, his chances to adjust are good. If, on the other hand, his family is such that it cannot satisfy his needs, he is likely to become vulnerable to frustration and to be easily enraged.

The same possibilities do exist for a placid baby, but it is probable that, because of his genetic inheritance, such an infant would not be so easily frustrated and may have a more tranquil babyhood. Later on in life, he may make fewer demands on his environment and may, in the long run, get along better. Is it possible, then, to explain Tom's difficulties on the basis of his early life experiences? Although there is no definite evidence, it is possible to assume that, given his inherited patterns, Tom's early needs for pleasure—such as his voracious appetite—were too much for his mother and that a conflict developed in the mother-child relationship very early in life. His unfortunate gastrointestinal difficulties seem to have added fuel to the fire because they conflicted with his mother's obsessive cleanliness, creating for him a vicious circle of frustrated appetite and unsatisfied needs, bad eating habits, and diarrhea. To these his mother reacted with disgust, by withdrawal of her affection, decreased interest in satisfying his needs, and finally total loss of interest in him. As this state of affairs worsened, Tom must have looked to others, craving affection and satisfaction of his frustrated wishes. This, of course, must have pleased his mother, who saw an opportunity to get rid of him.

Tom's father and grandmother, as we know, were the two people available to him from the beginning. The early loss of his father must have been a devastating blow. It was his father whom he sought when, confused and despairing, he was lying in the pit. His grandmother, on the other hand, took care of him for six years. She obviously liked the boy and must have provided him with love and some element of comfort, but again he was doomed to frustration. Her death, which he described so vividly to me, gave the picture of a pathetic little boy who suddenly was faced with the fear of the unknown and the certainty that life on earth was a miserable existence, interrupted only rarely by somewhat pleasant and short-lived interludes. These interludes involved an attempt to re-establish a close relationship with some other person on whom he could depend for support. At first he looked for these qualities in his wife, but was soon disappointed. He then established a relationship with the old woman who provided and cared for him. But it was his uncle who gave him the opportunity, during their drinking binges, to recapture a glimpse of his old relationship with his father, and it was the uncle's death that played an important role in triggering the first attack of Tom's ulcerative colitis. From then on, he tried valiantly to cope with the demands placed on him by the outside world, but he was too self-centered, too inexperienced, and too angry to succeed in his efforts to establish mature, meaningful relations with people. So he fought his battles alone and, as his frustrations increased, tried to drink himself to death, to kill himself, or at times, in fury and exasperation, to kill anyone who was in his way.

How much of all of this could have been prevented is a question that should be asked. But first one must specify what is meant by "all of this." From the results of the anaclitic treatment it is possible to say that Tom, despite his deprivations, early separations, and losses, was able to utilize his relationship with me therapeutically and to achieve some kind of modus vivendi. It can be argued, therefore, that if such an opportunity had been offered to him when he was a young child, or even in his early puberty, he might have been able to adjust more successfully during his adult life. What is most unfortunate is that he was unable to choose a wife who could have satisfied his many demands. Whether any wife could have satisfied Tom, when in addition she had to care for his children, is difficult to say. The fact that he made such extraordinary demands during the anaclitic treatment after being ill for so many years should not prove that he would have made equally unreasonable demands when he was first married. It must be remembered that Tom was willing to work hard and to provide for his family for a considerable period of time. Thus, from the psychological point of view, for any psychiatric steps to have been effective, they should have been taken during his childhood or possibly during his early adolescence.

One must not overlook the likelihood that Tom's psychological difficulties were due to some metabolic or biochemical defect which, if eliminated or corrected, would have resulted in the disappearance of his symptoms. This is possible, of course, as far as his ulcerative colitis was concerned. Going even further, it is also possible to imagine that eventually we shall be able to know all the biochemical reactions possible for the thinking and emotional processes, which are the functions of our brain. When this day comes, and it may not be too far away, we should still need to cope with individual reactions to early separations, losses, unforeseen complications of difficult mother-child relations, and the possible emotional trauma that may ensue. All our scientific knowledge, however, will not be able to uproot the idiosyncratic individualism of our personalities and the variations and novelties of our emotional and intellectual reactions, which, despite all the problems they can create, make life worth living.

There is no doubt that the anaclitic treatment presents formidable contraindications that make it impracticable for its routine use with other patients. I have already described the antagonism aroused in the nurses, caused by the great amount of strain placed upon them. Furthermore, other patients on the ward resented the lavish attention and privileges that were piled upon the "lucky patient," who in their eyes was receiving preferential treatment. This inequality among the patients caused repercussions on their own doctor-patient relationships. Three other patients requested that they receive anaclitic therapy while Tom was on our psychiatry ward. It was difficult for them to understand the explanations of their doctors, and they were annoyed when they were told they were "unsuitable" for such treatment.

Another disadvantage is that such therapy is very expensive, and only patients supported by funds from a grant or who are otherwise financially well-off can be treated in this way. The emotional demands placed upon the therapist are enormous and, as I have described, often actively interfere with the treatment process. Willingness and enthusiasm are not enough. Physical stamina is required when one has to be available to the patient "at all times." It could be said, of course, that the unrealistic satisfaction of all the patient's needs would be an impossibility if it were fully carried out with many patients. What, for instance, might one say if a patient asked for money or made other demands that could not be met? I was somewhat bothered by such an eventuality, but could reassure myself that Tom was regressing emotionally to a childlike or, better, infantlike state. Infants are not interested in money—they have simple needs. They want food and love. Food is easy to give. Love is a much more difficult thing to ask for from a therapist; but if he is able to respond with warmth and fondness for his patient, it will make all the difference in the world.

What was learned from the anaclitic relationship with Tom, then, was that at times much more is necessary than a simple doctor-patient relationship. When one is dealing with these basic and powerful early emotions that all of us have experienced but have been able more or less to master in our adult lives, ordinary therapeutic measures are not enough—basic and powerful methods are necessary. It is possible that our failure to treat successfully psychotic patients except on rare occasions results from our inability to meet the overwhelming demands that the patients make on their therapists. The most important thing about the experience with Tom was that anaclitic treatment saved his life. In a general hospital, therefore, where medicine and psychiatry work together, it is possible and at times advisable, with patients suffering from disabling psychological complications and psychosomatic illnesses, to try something drastic and new.

As far as anaclitic involvement is concerned, one may say that it is a closer relationship between patient and therapist than one usually encounters in psychotherapy or in psychoanalysis. The therapist does not simply attempt to win his patient's confidence and allow the transfer onto himself of the unconscious fantasies and emotional attitudes that are experienced by the patient concerning people in his past; nor does he simply help the patient regress to a dependent state. He must go beyond all these considerations. He must abandon temporarily his objective attitudes and attempt to encounter his patient on the patient's own level of existence and of primitive emotional functioning. The psychiatrist, contrary at times to his better judgment and to medical tradition, must give in to the patient's unrealistic demands. To a great extent he must rely on his own intuition and, on occasion, act against his own rational thinking and knowledge. At all times, despite these handicaps, he must also examine his own emotional reactions and acknowledge his own feelings, particularly when faced with constant requests for unending emotional support. He must forget his personal interests and responsibilities temporarily and try to get as close a glimpse as possible of his patient's behavior, despite irrational attacks and an endless bombardment of hostile projections. But, above all, he must observe and learn.

Throughout this time, the therapist feels unsure of himself—interested, yet annoyed; objective, yet irritated; helpful, yet at times helpless. But at the end, when he is able to witness the patient's ordeal and observe his battle against overpowering forces and drives, when he is able to realize to his own satisfaction the truths of earlier psychological observations that he has only read about, a transformation takes place within him. He feels that he also has emerged from some kind of pit—from a world of rigid compulsive attitudes, narrow-minded prejudices, and self-centered interests. He realizes that he has stripped himself of some of his own protective coverings and selfish wishes, that he is able to take a good look at himself. He suddenly feels freer; his thinking is simpler and more original; and he is even a trifle more humble as a person. For this, he remains forever grateful to his patient.

The anaclitic relationship, although it can be lifesaving to some patients in special circumstances, as it was for Tom, is not generally recommended as a practicable type of treatment for mental illness or ulcerative colitis. One wonders if it is a therapy at all. To those who want to observe and learn about emotional struggles, it may be of interest. To those, however, who want to look inside themselves and see themselves as they really are, thus becoming more tolerant of others and thereby better able to help their suffering patients, it is recommended as a unique and profound life experience.

DATE DUE

MAR 1 7 1983			
MAR 0 4 1983			